PLANT-BASED DIET COOKBOOK FOR BEGINNERS

DELICIOUS AND NUTRITIOUS RECIPES FOR LONG-TERM WELLNESS

Crystal Flynn

TABLE OF CONTENT

INTRODUCTION TO PLANT-BASED EATING

WHAT IS A PLANT-BASED DIET?

Transitioning to a plant-based diet involves centering your meals around whole, minimally processed plant foods. This means enjoying a diverse array of fruits, vegetables, grains, legumes, nuts, and seeds while minimizing or eliminating animal products. It's not about strict rules but rather about embracing a lifestyle that prioritizes the goodness of plants.

BENEFITS OF A PLANT-BASED LIFESTYLE

Adopting a plant-based lifestyle offers numerous health benefits. Research suggests that it can lower the risk of chronic diseases such as heart disease, diabetes, and certain cancers. Additionally, many individuals find that they achieve and maintain a healthy weight more easily on a plant-based diet, and experience increased energy levels and improved overall well-being. Beyond personal health, choosing plant-based options can have positive implications for the environment by reducing greenhouse gas emissions, conserving water, and preserving natural resources. Moreover, it aligns with ethical considerations by promoting compassion for animals and reducing their exploitation.

GETTING STARTED: ESSENTIAL INGREDIENTS AND EQUIPMENT

As you embark on your plant-based journey, it's essential to stock your kitchen with the right ingredients and equipment.

Begin by building a plant-based pantry stocked with essentials like whole grains (such as quinoa, brown rice, and oats), legumes (such as lentils, chickpeas, and black beans), a variety of spices and herbs, and plant-based condiments like nutritional yeast and tamari. Ensure your fridge is filled with a colorful assortment of fresh fruits and vegetables, and learn proper storage techniques to keep them fresh longer. Additionally, invest in basic kitchen tools such as a sharp chef's knife, cutting board, blender or food processor, pots and pans, and cooking utensils. With these essentials in place, you'll be well-equipped to explore the delicious world of plant-based cooking.

CHAPTER 1

BREAKFAST DELIGHTS

SMOOTHIE BOWLS AND BREAKFAST PARFAITS

SMOOTHIE BOWLS:

1. Choose your base: In a blender, combine your favorite fruits such as bananas, berries, mangoes, or pineapple with a liquid base like almond milk, coconut water, or yogurt.

2. Add a boost: Enhance your smoothie with nutritious add-ins such as spinach, kale, protein powder, or chia seeds for extra energy and satiety.

3. Blend until smooth: Blend all ingredients until smooth and creamy, adjusting the consistency as needed with additional liquid.

4. Pour into a bowl: Transfer the smoothie mixture into a bowl, then get creative with toppings such as sliced fruits, nuts, seeds, granola, coconut flakes, or drizzles of nut butter.

5. Enjoy: Grab a spoon and dig into your delicious and nourishing smoothie bowl for a refreshing start to your day.

BREAKFAST PARFAITS:

1. Layer your ingredients: Start by layering a glass or jar with a spoonful of yogurt, followed by a layer of granola or muesli, and then a layer of fresh fruits, bananas, berries, or mangoes.

2. Repeat: Continue layering yogurt, granola, and fruits until the glass or jar is filled to your liking,

ensuring to finish with a final layer of yogurt on top.

3. Garnish: Sprinkle additional toppings like nuts, seeds, or a drizzle of honey or maple syrup over the top layer of yogurt for added flavor and texture.

4. Serve chilled: Place the parfait in the refrigerator for at least 30 minutes to chill and allow the flavors to meld together.

5. Enjoy: Grab a spoon and savor each delicious layer of your breakfast parfait for a satisfying and nutritious morning treat.

1. Choose your oats: Select your preferred type of oats, whether it's old-fashioned rolled oats, quick oats, steel-cut oats, or instant oats.

2. Cook your oats: In a saucepan, combine oats with water or milk (such as almond milk, soy milk, or dairy milk) in a 2:1 ratio (2 parts liquid to 1 part oats).

3. Add flavor: Enhance your oatmeal with flavorings such as cinnamon, vanilla extract, or a pinch of salt for depth of flavor.

4. Customize: Get creative with your toppings by adding sliced fruits, nuts, seeds, nut butter, dried fruits, or sweeteners like honey or maple syrup.

5. Serve hot: Once your oatmeal reaches your desired consistency, transfer it to a bowl and top with your favorite toppings.

6. Enjoy: Grab a spoon and savor the comforting and nourishing goodness of your energizing morning oatmeal to kickstart your day with a nutritious boost.

SAVORY BREAKFAST OPTIONS:

1. Choose your base: Select your preferred savory base such as tofu, eggs, quinoa, or oats.

2. Prepare your ingredients: Chop vegetables like onions, bell peppers, spinach, tomatoes, mushrooms, or zucchini for added flavor and nutrition.

3. Cook your base: Depending on your choice of base, cook tofu scrambles, omelets, frittatas, or savory oatmeal according to your preferred method.

4. Add vegetables: Sautee or roast your chopped vegetables until tender, then add them to your

cooked base for an extra dose of vitamins and minerals.

5. Season to taste: Season your savory breakfast creation with herbs, spices, or condiments such as garlic powder, paprika, nutritional yeast, or hot sauce for added flavor.

6. Serve hot: Transfer your savory breakfast dish to a plate or bowl, then garnish with fresh herbs or additional toppings as desired.

7. Enjoy: Dive into your savory breakfast masterpiece and relish the savory flavors and textures that will tantalize your taste buds and keep you satisfied until your next meal.

CHAPTER 2

LUNCHTIME FAVORITES

HEARTY SALADS AND GRAIN BOWLS

HEARTY SALADS:

1. Choose your greens: Start with a base of leafy greens such as spinach, kale, arugula, or mixed salad greens.

2. Add protein: Incorporate protein-rich ingredients like grilled tofu, chickpeas, lentils, quinoa, or edamame to make your salad more filling and satisfying.

3. Load up on veggies: Layer your salad with a colorful assortment of fresh vegetables such as tomatoes, cucumbers, bell peppers, carrots, avocado, and radishes for added crunch and nutrition.

4. Enhance with toppings: Sprinkle your salad with toppings like nuts, seeds, dried fruits, crumbled cheese (if desired), or homemade croutons for texture and flavor.

5. Dress it up: Drizzle your salad with your favorite dressing or vinaigrette, or keep it simple with a squeeze of lemon juice and a drizzle of olive oil.

6. Toss and enjoy: Toss all the ingredients together until well combined, then transfer to a bowl or plate and enjoy your hearty and nutritious salad.

GRAIN BOWLS:

1. Choose your grain: Start with a base of cooked grains such as brown rice, quinoa, farro, barley, or couscous.

2. Add protein: Top your grain bowl with a plant-based protein source like tofu, tempeh, beans, lentils, or seitan for sustained energy and satiety.

3. Load up on veggies: Pile your grain bowl with a variety of cooked and raw vegetables such as roasted sweet potatoes, sautéed greens, steamed broccoli, cherry tomatoes, and sliced avocado for a colorful and nutritious meal.

4. Enhance with flavor: Add flavor and depth to your grain bowl with toppings like fresh herbs, toasted nuts or seeds, pickled vegetables, or a drizzle of tahini or plant-based yogurt sauce.

5. Mix it all: Mix all the ingredients in your bowl until well combined, then dig in and enjoy the satisfying and nourishing flavors of your grain bowl.

FLAVORFUL SANDWICHES AND WRAPS

SANDWICHES:

1. Choose your bread: Select your favorite type of bread, such as whole grain, ciabatta, sourdough, or pita.

2. Layer on the spreads: Spread your bread with condiments like hummus, avocado, pesto, mustard, or vegan mayo to add flavor and moisture to your sandwich.

3. Add protein: Layer your sandwich with protein-rich fillings such as sliced tofu, tempeh, vegan deli slices, or seitan for a satisfying meal.

4. Load up on veggies: Pack your sandwich with a variety of fresh vegetables like lettuce, spinach, cucumbers, tomatoes, bell peppers, onions, and sprouts for crunch and nutrition.

5. Finish with flavor: Add extra flavor and texture with toppings like sliced vegan cheese, pickles, olives, roasted red peppers, or sun-dried tomatoes.

6. Assemble and enjoy: Stack all the ingredients between your bread slices, then cut your sandwich in half and enjoy the delicious flavors and textures with every bite.

WRAPS:

1. Choose your wrap: Select your preferred type of wrap, such as whole grain, spinach, tomato, or gluten-free tortillas.

2. Spread on the sauce: Spread a thin layer of your favorite plant-based sauce or spread, like hummus, tzatziki, guacamole, or salsa, on the center of your wrap to add flavor and help hold the ingredients together.

3. Add protein: Layer your wrap with protein-rich fillings like tofu, tempeh, falafel, beans, or seitan for sustained energy and satiety.

4. Load up on veggies: Pile your wrap with a variety of fresh vegetables like lettuce, spinach, shredded carrots, cucumbers, bell peppers, avocado, and red cabbage for crunch and color.

5. Fold and roll: Fold the sides of your wrap inward, then tightly roll it up from the bottom to encase all the ingredients in a neat package.

6. Slice and enjoy: Slice your wrap in half diagonally, then serve and enjoy your flavorful and portable plant-based meal option!

SOUPS AND STEWS FOR A SATISFYING LUNCH

SOUPS:

1. Choose your base: Start with a flavorful plant-based broth or stock as the base of your soup, made with vegetables, mushrooms, or legumes.

2. Add vegetables: Add a variety of chopped vegetables like onions, carrots, celery, bell peppers, zucchini, and potatoes to the pot and simmer until tender.

3. Incorporate protein: Add plant-based protein sources like beans, lentils, tofu, tempeh, or seitan to make your soup more filling and satisfying.

4. Season to taste: Season your soup with herbs, spices, and aromatics like garlic, ginger, thyme, rosemary, cumin, or paprika for depth of flavor.

5. Simmer and serve: Let your soup simmer on the stove until all the flavors meld together, then ladle it into bowls and serve hot with your favorite toppings or accompaniments like crusty bread or crackers.

6. Enjoy: Sit back, relax, and enjoy the comforting and nourishing goodness of your homemade soup for a satisfying lunch that warms both body and soul.

1. Choose your protein: Select plant-based protein sources like tofu, tempeh, seitan, or legumes like lentils or chickpeas.

2. Brown the protein: Heat oil in a large pot or Dutch oven over medium heat, then brown your protein on all sides to develop flavor and texture.

3. Add aromatics: Add chopped onions, garlic, and other aromatics like carrots, celery, and bell peppers to the pot and sauté until softened and fragrant.

4. Incorporate liquid: Pour in your choice of plant-based liquid like vegetable broth, tomato sauce, or coconut milk to deglaze the pot and create a flavorful base for your stew.

5. Add vegetables: Add hearty vegetables like potatoes, sweet potatoes, squash, tomatoes, or root vegetables to the pot, along with herbs and spices for seasoning.

6. Simmer and stew: Let your stew simmer on the stove or in the oven until the protein is tender and the flavors

have melded together, stirring occasionally to prevent sticking.

7. Serve and enjoy: Ladle your hearty stew into bowls and serve hot, garnished with fresh herbs or a dollop of plant-based yogurt or sour cream if desired, and enjoy the hearty and satisfying flavors of your homemade creation.

CHAPTER 3

DINNER DAZZLERS

1. PLANT-POWERED PASTA DISHES

INGREDIENTS:

- Your favorite pasta (e.g., spaghetti, penne, fusilli)
- Assorted vegetables (e.g., bell peppers, zucchini, cherry tomatoes, spinach)
- Plant-based protein (e.g., tofu, tempeh, chickpeas)
- Olive oil
- Garlic
- Herbs and spices (e.g., basil, oregano, red pepper flakes)
- Vegan cheese (optional)
- Nutritional yeast (optional)
- Salt and pepper to taste

1. Cook pasta until al dente, following package directions.

2. Heat the olive oil in a large skillet over medium heat.

3. Add chopped vegetables to the skillet and cook until tender-crisp.

4. Incorporate your choice of plant-based protein (tofu, tempeh, chickpeas) into the skillet and cook until heated through.

5. Season with herbs and spices of your choice, such as basil, oregano, and red pepper flakes.

6. Add cooked pasta to the skillet and toss everything together until well combined.

7. Serve hot, garnished with vegan cheese or nutritional yeast if desired.

2. WHOLESOME STIR-FRIES AND CURRIES

INGREDIENTS:

- Assorted vegetables (e.g., broccoli, bell peppers, snap peas, carrots)
- Protein source (e.g., tofu, tempeh, seitan, edamame)
- Stir-fry sauce (e.g., soy sauce, teriyaki sauce, hoisin sauce)
- Aromatics (e.g., garlic, ginger, onion)
- Rice or noodles for serving
- Coconut milk or curry paste for curries
- Optional toppings (e.g., chopped peanuts, cilantro, green onions)

INSTRUCTIONS:

1. Set a big skillet or wok over medium-high heat and add the oil. Add minced garlic, ginger, and diced onion, and sauté until fragrant.

2. Add chopped vegetables to the skillet and stir-fry until they start to soften.

3. Add your choice of protein (tofu, tempeh, etc.) to the skillet and cook until lightly browned.

4. Pour in stir-fry sauce of your choice and toss everything together until well coated.

5. Serve stir-fry hot overcooked rice or noodles, and garnish with optional toppings if desired.

6. For curries, heat coconut milk or curry paste in a large pot over medium heat. Add chopped vegetables and protein, and simmer until everything is cooked through.

7. Serve curry hot over cooked rice, and garnish with optional toppings if desired.

3. CREATIVE VEGGIE-BASED MAIN COURSES

INGREDIENTS:

- Eggplant, portobello mushrooms, or cauliflower steaks
- Assorted vegetables (e.g., bell peppers, onions, tomatoes)
- Plant-based protein (e.g., lentils, beans, chickpeas)
- Herbs and spices (e.g., rosemary, thyme, paprika)
- Olive oil or vegetable broth for cooking
- Optional toppings (e.g., vegan cheese, breadcrumbs, fresh herbs)

INSTRUCTIONS:

1. Preheat the oven to 400°F (200°C). Slice eggplant, portobello mushrooms, or cauliflower into thick steaks.

2. Place vegetable steaks on a baking sheet lined with parchment paper. Drizzle with olive oil and add your favorite herbs and spices.

3. Roast vegetable steaks in the oven for 20-25 minutes, or until tender and lightly browned.

4. In a separate skillet, heat olive oil or vegetable broth over medium heat. Cook the chopped vegetables through.

5. Incorporate your choice of plant-based protein (lentils, beans, chickpeas) into the skillet and cook until heated through.

6. Season with additional herbs and spices as desired.

7. Serve roasted vegetable steaks hot with the vegetable and protein mixture on top, and garnish with optional toppings if desired.

CHAPTER 4

SNACK ATTACK

1. NUTRITIOUS SNACK IDEAS FOR ANYTIME

1. FRESH FRUIT:

Enjoy whole fruits like apples, bananas, berries, or oranges for a refreshing and naturally sweet snack.

Incorporating fresh fruit into your diet is a crucial aspect of maintaining optimal health. Fresh fruit is a rich source of essential vitamins and minerals, including vitamin C, potassium, and folate. These nutrients play a vital role in supporting immune function, healthy digestion, and overall well-being.

The antioxidant properties of fresh fruit also make it an effective tool in reducing the risk of chronic diseases such as heart disease, stroke, and certain cancers.

Additionally, the high fiber content in fresh fruit supports healthy digestion and can aid in weight management. Fresh fruit is a natural beauty booster, with its antioxidant and vitamin properties promoting healthy skin and supporting eye health. The cognitive benefits of fresh fruit are also noteworthy, with a diet rich in fruit shown to improve cognitive function and reduce the risk of age-related cognitive decline.

Incorporating a variety of fresh fruits into your vegetarian diet is a simple yet effective way to support overall health and well-being. Aim to include a rainbow of colors on your plate to ensure you're getting a range of nutrients and benefits.

2. RAW VEGGIES:

Dip baby carrots, celery sticks, cucumber slices, bell pepper strips, or cherry tomatoes in hummus or your favorite dip for a crunchy and satisfying snack.

As a vegetarian, incorporating raw vegetables into your diet is a great way to boost your overall health and well-being. Raw vegetables are packed with vital nutrients, enzymes, and antioxidants that are often lost during cooking. By eating them in their natural state, you can reap numerous benefits, including increased nutrient absorption, improved digestion, boosted energy, enhanced immune function, weight management, glowing skin, reduced inflammation, and support for eye health.

Raw vegetables contain higher levels of vitamins, minerals, and antioxidants than their cooked counterparts, and are rich in fiber, which helps promote healthy digestion and support the growth of beneficial gut bacteria. The antioxidants and phytochemicals in raw vegetables also help protect your cells from damage, reduce inflammation, and support immune function.

Raw vegetables are low in calories, high in fiber, and rich in water content, making them an excellent addition to a weight management plan. The antioxidants and vitamins in raw vegetables also help protect your skin from damage, promote collagen production, and give you a radiant glow. Incorporating raw vegetables into your vegetarian diet is a simple and delicious way to unlock a world of plant-based possibilities and support your overall health and well-being.

3. **NUTS AND SEEDS**:

 Snack on a handful of almonds, walnuts, pumpkin seeds, or sunflower seeds for a dose of healthy fats and protein.

Nuts and seeds are a nutritious and versatile addition to a plant-based diet, offering a wealth of health benefits and culinary possibilities. These tiny powerhouses are packed with protein, healthy fats, fiber, vitamins, and minerals, making them an excellent snack or ingredient to enhance your meals.

Eating nuts and seeds can help lower cholesterol and triglycerides, improve heart health, and support weight management. They are also rich in antioxidants and anti-inflammatory compounds, which can help protect against chronic diseases such as cancer, diabetes, and cognitive decline.

Some benefits of nuts and seeds include:
- Protein power: Many nuts and seeds are high in protein, making them an excellent option for vegetarians and vegans.

- Healthy fats: Nuts and seeds contain healthy fats that support heart health and satisfy hunger.
- Fiber boost: Nuts and seeds are rich in fiber, which supports healthy digestion and satiety.
- Vitamins and minerals: Nuts and seeds are a good source of essential vitamins and minerals like magnesium, selenium, and zinc.
- Antioxidant-rich: Nuts and seeds contain antioxidants that help protect against cell damage and inflammation.
- Supports heart health: Eating nuts and seeds regularly can help lower cholesterol and triglycerides, reducing the risk of heart disease.

Other popular nuts and seeds to include in your plant-based diet are:

- Almonds
- Walnuts
- Chia seeds
- Flaxseeds
- Pumpkin seeds
- Sunflower seeds
- Hemp seeds
- Cashews
- Pistachios

Enjoy nuts and seeds as a snack, add them to your oatmeal or yogurt, or use them as a topping for salads and stir-fries. With their rich nutritional profile and versatility, nuts and seeds are a great addition to a healthy and delicious plant-based diet.

Opt for plain Greek yogurt and top it with granola, sliced fruits, or a drizzle of honey for a creamy and protein-packed snack.

Greek yogurt is a nutritious and versatile addition to a plant-based diet, offering a wealth of health benefits and culinary possibilities. Made from soy or coconut milk, Greek yogurt is a great alternative to traditional dairy yogurt, providing a similar texture and taste without animal products. This creamy delight is packed with protein, calcium, and probiotics, making it an excellent snack or ingredient to enhance your meals.

Eating Greek yogurt can help support digestive health, boost the immune system, and aid in weight management. The probiotics in Greek yogurt help maintain a healthy gut microbiome, supporting the absorption of nutrients and reducing symptoms of irritable bowel syndrome. Additionally, Greek yogurt is a good source of protein, making it an excellent option for vegetarians and vegans looking to increase their protein intake.

Some of the key benefits of Greek yogurt include:

- High in protein
- Rich in calcium
- Packed with probiotics
- Supports digestive health
- Boosts immune system
- Aids in weight management

Enjoy Greek yogurt as a snack, add it to your oatmeal or smoothies, or use it as a base for salad dressings and dips. With its rich nutritional profile and versatility, Greek yogurt is a great addition to a healthy and delicious plant-based diet.

5. RICE CAKES:

Spread almond butter or avocado on rice cakes and top with sliced bananas or strawberries for a satisfying and crunchy snack.

Rice cakes are a popular snack that has been enjoyed for centuries in many Asian cultures. Made from rice flour and water, these crispy treats are not only delicious but also packed with nutrients and health benefits. Rice cakes are a great option for those with gluten intolerance or celiac disease, as they are gluten-free. With approximately 120-150 calories per serving, rice cakes are a great snack for weight management.
They are also high in fiber, supporting healthy digestion, bowel function, and satiety. Rice cakes are a good source of essential minerals like manganese, selenium, and magnesium, crucial for maintaining overall health. They contain antioxidants that help protect the body against free radicals and oxidative and support healthy gut bacteria.

Rice cakes can be enjoyed in various ways, such as topped with avocado, hummus, or peanut butter, or used as a base for mini sandwiches. They can also be seasoned with herbs and spices for added flavor. With their crunchy texture and nutty flavor, rice cakes are a satisfying snack that can be enjoyed guilt-free.

6. POPCORN:

Air-pop popcorn and season it with nutritional yeast, cinnamon, or chili powder for a flavorful and low-calorie snack option.

Popcorn is a beloved snack that's not only tasty but also packed with nutrients and health benefits. This whole grain food is made from corn kernels that "pop" when heated, resulting in a crispy and fluffy treat. Popcorn is a good source of dietary fiber, supporting healthy digestion and bowel function. It contains antioxidants, which protect the body from free radicals and oxidative stress. As a whole-grain food, popcorn is a great source of essential nutrients like vitamins, minerals, and phytochemicals. Air-popped popcorn is a low-calorie snack, with approximately 30 calories per cup.

Popcorn can be enjoyed as a healthy snack by choosing air-popped or microwave options without added salt or oil. You can also season it with herbs and spices for added flavor. With its crunchy texture and nutty flavor, popcorn is a satisfying snack that's perfect for movie nights or anytime munching.

7. EDAMAME:

Enjoy steamed edamame sprinkled with sea salt for a protein-rich and satisfying snack.

Edamame, also known as soybeans, is a type of legume that's packed with nutrients and health benefits. These small, green pods are a staple in Asian cuisine and are often served boiled or steamed as a snack or appetizer.

Edamame is an excellent source of protein, fiber, and vitamins, making it a great option for vegetarians and vegans. It's also rich in antioxidants and phytochemicals, which have been shown to reduce the risk of chronic diseases like heart disease, diabetes, and certain cancers.

Edamame is high in dietary fiber, supporting healthy digestion and bowel function. It contains antioxidants and phytochemicals that help protect the body against free radicals and oxidative stress.

Edamame is low in calories, with approximately 125 calories per 1/2 cup serving. Nutritional Information (per serving): Calories: 125, Fat: 2g, Carbohydrates: 10g, Fiber: 5g, Protein: 10g. Enjoy edamame as a healthy snack by steaming or boiling them, or adding them to stir-fries and salads. With its nutty flavor and crunchy texture, edamame is a delicious and nutritious addition to any meal!

2. HOMEMADE DIPS AND SPREADS

1. HUMMUS:

Blend chickpeas, tahini, lemon juice, garlic, and olive oil until smooth and creamy for a classic and versatile dip.

Hummus, a popular Middle Eastern dip or spread made from chickpeas, tahini, garlic, and lemon juice, is a tasty and healthy addition to any meal. With its creamy texture and nutty flavor, hummus is not only delicious but also packed with nutrients and health benefits. It's an excellent source of plant-based protein, fiber, and healthy fats, making it a great option for vegetarians and vegans.

Hummus also contains antioxidants, vitamins, and minerals like vitamin C, vitamin E, calcium, and phosphorus, which support overall health and well-being. Enjoy hummus as a healthy dip for vegetables, crackers, or pita bread, or use it as a spread for sandwiches and wraps. With its numerous health benefits and delicious taste, hummus is a perfect addition to a healthy and balanced diet. Nutritional Information (per serving): Calories: 100, Fat: 10g, Carbohydrates: 10g, Fiber: 5g, Protein: 5g.

2. GUACAMOLE:

Mash ripe avocados with lime juice, diced tomatoes, onions, cilantro, and a pinch of salt for a creamy and flavorful dip.

Guacamole, a popular Mexican dip made from avocados, lime juice, and spices, is a delicious and healthy addition to any meal. With its creamy texture and rich flavor, guacamole is not only a tasty dip for vegetables, chips, and crackers but also packed with nutrients and health benefits. Avocados, the main ingredient in guacamole, are a rich source of healthy fats, fiber, and various vitamins and minerals like potassium, vitamin C, and vitamin E.

Guacamole also contains antioxidants and phytochemicals that help protect against cell damage and oxidative stress. Enjoy guacamole as a healthy dip or spread, or use it as a topping for salads, sandwiches, and grilled meats. With its numerous health benefits and delicious taste, guacamole is a perfect addition to a healthy and balanced diet.

3. SALSA:

Combine diced tomatoes, onions, jalapenos, cilantro, lime juice, and salt for a fresh and zesty dip that pairs well with chips or veggies.

Salsa, a popular Mexican condiment made from tomatoes, onions, jalapenos, and cilantro, is a flavorful and healthy addition to any meal. With its spicy kick and tangy flavor, salsa is not only a great topping for tacos, grilled meats, and vegetables but also packed with nutrients and health benefits. Tomatoes, the main ingredient in salsa, are rich in vitamin C, lycopene, and potassium, which support heart health, immune function, and anti-inflammatory effects. The onions in salsa contain fiber, vitamin C, and various antioxidants, while the jalapenos add a boost of vitamin C and capsaicin, which has natural pain-relieving properties. Cilantro, also known as coriander, contains antioxidants and phytochemicals that help protect against cell damage and oxidative stress.

Salsa is also low in calories and fat, making it a great alternative to mayonnaise or sour cream. Enjoy salsa as a healthy condiment or dip, or use it as a topping for salads, sandwiches, and grilled meats. With its numerous health benefits and delicious taste, salsa is a perfect addition to a healthy and balanced diet.

Salsa also offers several health benefits. The antioxidants and phytochemicals in salsa may help reduce the risk of chronic diseases like heart disease, diabetes, and certain cancers. The capsaicin in jalapenos may also help alleviate symptoms of arthritis and other inflammatory conditions.

Salsa is a flavorful and nutritious condiment that can add excitement and health benefits to any meal. So go ahead, add some salsa to your favorite dishes, and enjoy the taste and nutritional benefits.

4. BABA GANOUSH:

Roast eggplant until soft, then blend it with tahini, garlic, lemon juice, and olive oil for a smoky and savory dip. Baba Ganoosh, a beloved Middle Eastern dip, offers a multitude of health benefits, making it a nutritious addition to your culinary journey. With its rich blend of antioxidants from eggplants, tahini, garlic, and lemon juice, Baba Ganoosh shields cells from damage and reduces inflammation, supporting overall health. The healthy fats in tahini and eggplants also support heart well-being by lowering cholesterol levels and improving blood vessel function.

The fiber-rich eggplants and tahini regulate bowel movements and prevent constipation. Phytochemicals in Baba Ganoosh may reduce inflammation, promoting overall well-being, while tahini's calcium content supports strong bones. Garlic's compounds enhance immune function, and eggplants' potassium content helps alleviate anxiety and stress. Indulge in Baba Ganoosh, a delicious and nutritious delight that nourishes both body and taste buds.

5. TZATZIKI:

Mix Greek yogurt with grated cucumber, garlic, dill, lemon juice, and salt for a creamy and refreshing dip that's perfect with pita chips or veggies.

Tzatziki, a beloved Greek condiment made from yogurt, cucumbers, garlic, and dill, is a tangy and refreshing addition to your plant-based journey. With its high water content and cooling flavor, Tzatziki helps hydrate and soothe the body, making it perfect for hot summer days and gatherings. The yogurt provides a boost of protein and calcium, supporting strong bones and muscles, while the cucumbers add antioxidants and anti-inflammatory properties, reducing the risk of chronic diseases. Garlic enhances immune function and reduces inflammation, and dill provides additional antioxidants and digestive benefits, supporting a healthy gut.

Enjoy Tzatziki as a dip for vegetables, a sauce for grilled portobello mushrooms or eggplant, or a side dish for salads and sandwiches. This versatile condiment is not only delicious but also packed with nutrients, making it a great addition to a healthy and balanced plant-based diet.

6. PESTO:

Blend fresh basil leaves, garlic, pine nuts, Parmesan cheese (or nutritional yeast for a vegan option), and olive oil until smooth for a vibrant and flavorful spread

Pesto, a classic Italian sauce made from basil, garlic, pine nuts, Parmesan cheese, and olive oil, is a flavorful and nutritious addition to your plant-based journey. With its vibrant green color and rich aroma, Pesto adds a burst of flavor to pasta dishes, salads, and sandwiches. Basil provides antioxidants and anti-inflammatory properties, while garlic enhances immune function and reduces inflammation. Pine nuts offer healthy fats and protein, and olive oil provides additional antioxidants and heart-healthy benefits.

Enjoy Pesto as a sauce for whole-grain pasta, a dip for vegetables, or a spread for sandwiches. This versatile sauce is not only delicious but also packed with nutrients, making it a great addition to a healthy and balanced plant-based diet.

Note: For a plant-based version of Pesto, you can replace Parmesan cheese with nutritional yeast or another vegan alternative.

7. NUT BUTTER:

Make your nut butter by blending roasted nuts (such as almonds, peanuts, or cashews) with a touch of salt and optional sweetener until creamy for a delicious and protein-rich spread.

Nut Butter, a delicious and versatile spread made from a diverse range of nuts and seeds, is a tasty and nutritious addition to your plant-based journey. With its creamy texture and rich flavor, Nut Butter is perfect for sandwiches, smoothies, baking, snacking, and even savory dishes. Whether you prefer classic peanut butter, almond butter, cashew butter, sunflower seed butter, soy butter, coconut butter, or another variety, Nut Butter is a great way to add healthy fats, protein, fiber, and essential vitamins and minerals to your diet.

Nuts and seeds are packed with antioxidants, anti-inflammatory properties, and a range of essential nutrients, making Nut Butter a nutritious choice for those looking to fuel their bodies with whole foods. Enjoy Nut Butter as a spread on whole-grain toast, a dip for fresh fruit, an ingredient in your favorite smoothie or energy ball recipe, or as a creamy addition to your favorite dishes, such as curries, stir-fries, or sauces.

With its versatility and nutritional benefits, Nut Butter is a great addition to a healthy and balanced plant-based diet. Whether you're a fan of creamy peanut butter or prefer the nutty flavor of cashew butter, there's a Nut

Butter out there for everyone. So go ahead, spread it on thick, and enjoy the delicious taste and nutritional benefits of Nut Butter!

3. SWEET AND SAVORY BITES

1. ENERGY BALLS:

Combine dates, nuts, seeds, oats, and your favorite mix-ins like chocolate chips or dried fruits in a food processor, then roll into bite-sized balls for a nutritious and portable snack.

Energy Balls, a popular snack made from a combination of nut butter, oats, and honey, are a tasty and nutritious addition to your plant-based journey. These bite-sized balls of energy are perfect for snacking on the go, post-workout fueling, or as a healthy treat for kids and adults alike.

With their rich blend of nut butter, oats, and honey, Energy Balls provide sustained energy, healthy fats, protein, and fiber, making them an excellent choice for a quick pick-me-up or a pre-workout snack. Nut butter offers antioxidants and anti-inflammatory properties, while oats provide additional fiber and a range of essential vitamins and minerals, including iron, zinc, and potassium. Honey adds natural sweetness and antimicrobial properties, making it a great alternative to refined sugars.

Energy Balls are also incredibly versatile, allowing you to customize them to your taste preferences and dietary needs.

Some popular variations include:

- Adding chocolate chips or cocoa powder for a sweet treat
- Using different types of nut butter, such as peanut butter, cashew butter, or almond butter
- Adding in seeds, like chia, flax, or hemp, for extra nutrition and crunch
- Using coconut flakes or shredded coconut for added texture and flavor
- Making them with different types of milk, like almond, soy, or coconut milk
- Adding in dried fruits, like cranberries or raisins, for natural sweetness and chewiness

Energy Balls are also a great way to get creative with your nutrition, allowing you to experiment with different ingredients and flavors to find your favorite combination. Plus, they're easy to make in large batches, making them a convenient snack for meal prep or on-the-go fueling.

Whether you're a busy professional, an athlete, or a parent looking for a healthy snack option, Energy Balls are a great choice. They're easy to make, fun to eat, and packed with nutrients, making them a great addition to a healthy and balanced plant-based diet. So why not give them a try and experience the energy-boosting benefits for yourself?

2. VEGGIE STICKS WITH DIP:

Serve sliced cucumbers, carrots, bell peppers, and celery with hummus, guacamole, or tzatziki for a satisfying and crunchy snack.

Veggie Sticks with Dip, a classic snack combination, is a tasty and nutritious addition to your plant-based journey. Crunchy veggie sticks paired with a creamy dip make for a satisfying snack that's perfect for munching on the go, as a side dish, or as a healthy alternative to chips and dip.

Veggie sticks, such as carrots, cucumbers, bell peppers, cherry tomatoes, and many more, provide a burst of essential vitamins, minerals, and antioxidants, making them a great way to fuel your body with whole foods. Each veggie stick offers its unique nutritional benefits, ranging from vitamin A-rich carrots to hydrating cucumbers and antioxidant-packed bell peppers.

The dip adds a creamy and flavorful element, with options like hummus, guacamole, ranch, tzatziki, and many more. Each dip offers its nutritional benefits, such as the protein and fiber in hummus, the healthy fats in guacamole, and the probiotics in ranch.

Enjoy Veggie Sticks with Dip as a:
- Quick snack to curb hunger and boost energy
- Side dish for meals, adding crunch and flavor
- Healthy alternative to chips and dip, satisfying your cravings
- Crunchy addition to salads or wraps, adding texture and flavor
- Fun and easy snack for kids and adults alike, promoting healthy eating habits

Some popular veggie stick and dip combinations include:

- Carrot and celery sticks with hummus
- Cucumber slices with dill dip
- Bell pepper strips with guacamole
- Cherry tomatoes with ranch dip
- Radish slices with French onion dip

Feel free to get creative with your veggie stick and dip choices, experimenting with different combinations to find your favorite pairings. With the versatility of veggie sticks and dips, the possibilities are endless! Enjoy the crunchy, delicious, and nutritious benefits of this plant-based snack, perfect for a healthy and balanced lifestyle.

3. CHEESE AND CRACKERS:

Pair whole grain crackers with sliced cheese, grapes, and nuts for a simple and satisfying snack. Vegan Cheese and Crackers, a classic snack combination, gets a plant-based twist! Enjoy the creamy taste of vegan cheese paired with the crunch of whole-grain crackers, perfect for a quick snack or as a side dish.

Vegan cheese alternatives, made from nuts, seeds, or soy, offer a similar taste and texture to traditional cheese, without the dairy. Choose from a variety of flavors like cheddar, mozzarella, or feta, each with its unique taste profile.

Pair your vegan cheese with whole-grain crackers, made from ingredients like oats, quinoa, or brown rice, for a satisfying crunch. Look for crackers with minimal added ingredients and no artificial preservatives.

Enjoy Vegan Cheese and Crackers as a:

- Quick snack to curb hunger and boost energy
- Side dish for meals, adding flavor and texture
- Healthy alternative to traditional cheese and crackers
- Satisfying crunch for veggie sticks or fruit
- Fun and easy snack for kids and adults alike

Some popular vegan cheese and cracker combinations include:
- Vegan cheddar with oat crackers
- Vegan mozzarella with whole-grain breadsticks
- Vegan feta with olive oil crackers
- Vegan cream cheese with whole-grain bagel chips

Get creative with your vegan cheese and cracker choices, exploring different flavors and pairings. Enjoy the delicious and satisfying benefits of this plant-based snack!

4. STUFFED DATES:

Fill pitted dates with almond butter, cream cheese, or goat cheese, then sprinkle with sea salt or chopped nuts for a sweet and savory treat.

Stuffed Dates, a tasty and versatile snack, are a great addition to your plant-based journey, offering a perfect blend of natural sweetness and savory flavors. Sweet and succulent dates filled with a variety of ingredients like nuts, seeds, cheese alternatives, and fresh herbs make for a delightful treat that's not only delicious but also packed with nutrients.

Dates, a natural source of sweetness, provide a boost of potassium, fiber, and antioxidants, making them an excellent choice for a healthy snack. By stuffing them with a range of ingredients, you can create a snack that's both sweet and savory, satisfying your cravings while nourishing your body.

Some popular ingredients to stuff dates with include:
- Crunchy nuts like almonds, walnuts, or pecans, adding healthy fats and protein

- Seeds like pumpkin, chia, or sunflower, provide additional fiber and nutrients
- Vegan cheese alternatives like cream cheese or goat cheese, offer a tangy and creamy element
- Fresh herbs like parsley, rosemary, or thyme, adding a burst of flavor and antioxidants

Enjoy Stuffed Dates as a:

- Healthy snack on their own, perfect for curbing hunger and boosting energy
- Addition to salads or bowls, adding natural sweetness and texture
- Sweet and savory side dish, complementing a variety of meals
- Appetizer or tapas option, ideal for social gatherings and events
- Delicious topping for oatmeal, yogurt, or ice cream, adding flavor and nutrition

Some popular stuffed date combinations include:

- Almond and cream cheese stuffed dates, a classic sweet and savory pairing

- Walnut and chia seed stuffed dates, a crunchy and
nutritious option
- Pumpkin seed and rosemary stuffed dates, a flavorful
and herby combination
- Goat cheese alternative and parsley stuffed dates, a
tangy and fresh twist

Get creative with your stuffed date fillings and enjoy the
sweet and savory benefits of this plant-based snack,
perfect for a healthy and balanced lifestyle.

5. RICE PAPER ROLLS:

Fill rice paper wrappers with thinly sliced veggies, tofu, fresh herbs, and vermicelli noodles, then dip in a flavorful sauce for a light and refreshing snack.

Rice Paper Rolls, a popular Vietnamese snack, are a tasty and healthy addition to your plant-based journey, offering a perfect blend of flavors, textures, and nutrients. Thin rice paper wrappers filled with a variety of ingredients like vegetables, herbs, nuts, and fruits make for a delicious and refreshing treat that's not only delicious but also packed with health benefits.

Rice paper, made from rice flour and water, is a gluten-free and low-calorie alternative to traditional wraps, making it an excellent option for those with dietary restrictions or preferences. The fillings offer a range of flavors and textures, from crunchy vegetables to sweet and tangy fruits, and protein-rich nuts to fresh and fragrant herbs.

Enjoy Rice Paper Rolls as a:

- Healthy snack on their own, perfect for curbing hunger and boosting energy
- Side dish for meals, adding flavor and nutrition to your plate
- Appetizer or tapas option, ideal for social gatherings and events
- Refreshing summer treat, perfect for hot days and outdoor activities
- Fun and easy snack for kids and adults alike, promoting healthy eating habits

Some popular rice paper roll combinations include:

- Veggie delight: carrots, cucumbers, bell peppers, and mint
- Fruit and nut: mango, pineapple, peanuts, and cilantro
- Protein-packed: tofu, avocado, sprouts, and cashews
- Spicy kick: cucumber, bell peppers, jalapeño, and cilantro
- Mediterranean twist: hummus, tabbouleh, feta, and olives

Get creative with your rice paper roll fillings and enjoy the delicious and refreshing benefits of this plant-based snack, perfect for a healthy and balanced lifestyle. Experiment with different ingredients and flavors to find your favorite combinations, and enjoy the versatility and nutrition of Rice Paper Rolls!

6. APPLE SLICES WITH NUT BUTTER:

Spread almond butter or peanut butter on apple slices and top with granola or dried fruits for a sweet and satisfying snack.

Apple Slices with Nut Butter, a classic snack combination, is a tasty and healthy addition to your plant-based journey, offering a perfect blend of flavors, textures, and nutrients. Crunchy apple slices paired with creamy nut butter make for a satisfying snack that's perfect for any time of day, whether you're looking for a quick energy boost, a healthy side dish, or a delicious treat.

Apples, a rich source of fiber, vitamins, and antioxidants, provide a delicious and healthy base for this snack. With various types to choose from, like Granny Smith, Honeycrisp, Fuji, and Gala, you can mix and match to find your favorite combination. Apples offer numerous health benefits, including:

- Fiber-rich contents to support digestive health and promote satiety
- Antioxidants to protect against chronic diseases like heart disease, diabetes, and certain cancers
- Vitamin C for immune system support and collagen production
- Low-calorie count for weight management and reduced risk of obesity

Pairing apples with nut butter takes this snack to the next level. Nut butter, made from nuts like peanuts, almonds, cashews, or sunflower seeds, provides:

- Brain function and long-lasting energy from healthy fats
- Protein for muscle recovery and growth

- Fiber to support digestive health and promote satiety
- Antioxidants to protect against chronic diseases
- Magnesium and potassium for heart health and blood pressure management

Enjoy Apple Slices with Nut Butter as a:

- Quick snack to curb hunger and boost energy
- Healthy side dish for meals or as a topping for oatmeal or yogurt
- After-school snacks for kids, promoting healthy eating habits, and supporting growth and development
- Post-workout snack, providing protein and healthy fats for muscle recovery and growth
- Delicious and satisfying treat any time of day, supporting mental health and well-being

Some popular nut butter and apple combinations include:

- Classic peanut butter and Granny Smith apples
- Creamy almond butter and Honeycrisp apples
- Crunchy cashew butter and Fuji apples
- Smooth sunflower seed butter and Gala apples

Get creative with your nut butter and apple pairings and enjoy the delicious and nutritious benefits of this plant-based snack, perfect for a healthy and balanced lifestyle.

Try different types of nuts and apples to find your favorite combinations and enjoy the versatility and nutrition of Apple Slices with Nut Butter.

7. POPCORN TRAIL MIX:

Combine air-popped popcorn with nuts, seeds, dried fruits, and a sprinkle of cinnamon or cocoa powder for a crunchy and flavorful snack mix.

Popcorn trail mix is a satisfying snack that combines the crunchy texture of popcorn with the nutty flavor of nuts and seeds. This tasty mix is perfect for movie nights, on-the-go snacking, or as a healthy addition to your lunch or breakfast routine. With its versatile flavor profile, popcorn trail mix can be customized to suit any taste preference, from sweet and salty to savory and spicy.

But what sets popcorn trail mix apart is its impressive nutritional profile. This snack is packed with a range of beneficial nutrients that can support overall health and well-being.

Here are some of the key health benefits of popcorn trail mix:

- Whole Grain Goodness: Popcorn is a whole grain that provides sustained energy, fiber, and essential vitamins and minerals.

- Protein Power: Nuts and seeds in popcorn trail mix deliver a boost of protein to support muscle growth and repair, making it an excellent snack for fitness enthusiasts and individuals with busy lifestyles.

- Antioxidant Boost: Dried fruits, nuts, and seeds in popcorn trail mix are rich in antioxidants, which help protect cells from damage caused by free radicals. This can lead to reduced inflammation, improved skin health, and a lower risk of chronic diseases.

-Healthy Fats: Nuts and seeds in popcorn trail mix provide healthy fats that support heart health, brain function, and the absorption of essential vitamins and minerals.

- Fiber-Rich: Popcorn trail mix is a good source of dietary fiber, which supports healthy digestion, prevents constipation, and can help manage blood sugar levels

-Low in Calories: When made with wholesome ingredients, popcorn trail mix can be a low-calorie snack option that supports weight management and reduces the risk of chronic diseases.

By incorporating popcorn trail mix into your diet, you can enjoy a delicious and nutritious snack that supports your overall health and well-being.

CHAPTER 5

SIDE DISHES TO IMPRESS

1. VIBRANT VEGETABLE SIDES

1. ROASTED BRUSSELS SPROUTS:

Toss halved Brussels sprouts with olive oil, salt, and pepper, then roast in the oven until caramelized and crispy for a flavorful and nutritious side dish.

Here's a step-by-step guide on how to cook them:

Ingredients:

- 1 pound Brussels sprouts, halved

- 2 tablespoons olive oil

- Salt and pepper, to taste

- (Optional): You can enhance the flavor with garlic powder, paprika, or any other seasonings that you prefer.

Instructions:

1. Preheat your oven to 400°F (200°C).

2. In a large bowl, toss the halved Brussels sprouts with olive oil, salt, and pepper until they're evenly coated.

3. If desired, add garlic powder, paprika, or other seasonings and toss to combine.

4. Arrange the Brussels sprouts evenly on a baking sheet.

5. Roast in the preheated oven for 20-25 minutes, or until the Brussels sprouts are:

- Caramelized: dark brown and sticky on the outside

- Crispy: tender on the inside, with a satisfying crunch on the outside

6. Remove from the oven and serve hot.

Tips:

- Cut off any damaged or discolored leaves from the Brussels sprouts before halving them.

- If using garlic powder or paprika, start with a small amount (about 1/4 teaspoon) and adjust to taste.

- To enhance the caramelization process, you can increase the oven temperature to 425°F (220°C) for the last 5-7 minutes of roasting. Pay close attention to them to prevent overcooking!

- Roasted Brussels sprouts are a great side dish for many plant-based meals.

Roasted Brussels sprouts are a tasty and nutritious vegetable dish that offers several health benefits. As a cruciferous vegetable, Brussels sprouts are rich in vitamins, minerals, and antioxidants that support overall health and well-being.

Here are some of the key health benefits of roasted Brussels sprouts:

- Good Source of Vitamins and Minerals: Roasted Brussels sprouts are a good source of vitamins C and K, folate, and fiber.

- Antioxidant-Rich: Brussels sprouts contain a range of antioxidants that help protect cells from damage.

- Supports Healthy Digestion: The fiber content in Brussels sprouts can help promote healthy digestion and prevent constipation.

- May Support Heart Health: The fiber, vitamins, and antioxidants in Brussels sprouts may help support heart health.

- Nutritious and Low in Calories: Roasted Brussels sprouts are a low-calorie, nutrient-dense food that can be a healthy addition to a balanced diet.

By incorporating roasted Brussels sprouts into your diet, you can enjoy a delicious and nutritious side dish that supports your overall health and well-being.

2. GARLIC GREEN BEANS:

 Sautee trimmed green beans with minced garlic, olive oil, and a splash of soy sauce until tender-crisp and fragrant for a simple yet delicious side.

Here's a step-by-step guide on how to cook them:

Ingredients:
- 1 pound fresh green beans, trimmed
- 2 cloves garlic, minced
- 2 tablespoons olive oil
- 1 tablespoon of soy sauce (or tamari for those who prefer a gluten-free option)

- (Optional): lemon wedges or zest for added brightness

Instructions:

1. Warm up the olive oil in a spacious skillet or wok on medium-high heat.
2. Add the minced garlic and sauté for 1-2 minutes, until fragrant.
3. Add the trimmed green beans and sauté for 3-5 minutes, until they start to soften.
4. Pour in the soy sauce and continue cooking for another 2-3 minutes, until the green beans are tender-crisp.
5. Season with salt and pepper to taste.
6. Serve hot, garnished with lemon wedges or zest if desired.

Tips:

- Use fresh, bright green beans for the best flavor and texture.
- Feel free to customize the amount of garlic to suit your personal preference.
- If using lemon, squeeze a slice over the green beans for a burst of citrus flavor.

- Garlic green beans pair well with many plant-based main dishes.

Garlic green beans are a flavorful and nutritious vegetable dish that combines the health benefits of green beans with the added benefits of garlic. Green beans are a low-calorie, nutrient-dense food that is rich in vitamins, minerals, and antioxidants. Garlic, on the other hand, contains compounds that have antibacterial, antiviral, and antifungal properties.

Here are some of the key health benefits of garlic green beans:

- Low in Calories: Garlic green beans are a low-calorie food that can help support weight management.

- Rich in Vitamins and Minerals: Green beans are a good source of vitamins C and K, potassium, and fiber.

- Antioxidant-Rich: Green beans contain antioxidants that help protect cells from damage.

- Supports Healthy Digestion: The fiber content in green beans can help promote healthy digestion and prevent constipation.

- May Help Lower Cholesterol: The fiber, vitamins, and antioxidants in garlic green beans may help support heart health.

- Nutritious and Delicious: Garlic green beans are a tasty and nutritious side dish that can add flavor and nutrition to a variety of meals.

By incorporating garlic green beans into your diet, you can enjoy a delicious and nutritious vegetable dish that supports your overall health and well-being.

3. HONEY GLAZED CARROTS:

Roast whole carrots tossed in honey, butter, and thyme until tender and caramelized for a sweet and savory side that's sure to impress.

Here's a step-by-step guide on how to cook them:

Ingredients:
- 4-6 whole carrots, peeled
- 2 tablespoons honey
- 1 tablespoon butter
- 2 sprigs fresh thyme
- Salt and pepper, to taste

Instructions:
1. Preheat your oven to 425°F (220°C).
2. In a large bowl, whisk together honey, butter, and thyme until well combined.
3. Add the peeled carrots and toss to coat them evenly with the honey glaze.
4. Season with salt and pepper to taste.
5. Spread the carrots in a single layer on a baking sheet.
6. Roast in the preheated oven for 25-30 minutes, or until the carrots are:

- Tender: easily pierced with a fork

- Caramelized: golden brown and sticky on the outside

7. Remove from the oven and serve hot.

Tips:

- Use high-quality honey for the best flavor.

- Adjust the amount of thyme to your taste.

- To enhance the caramelization process, increase the oven temperature to 450°F (230°C) for the last 5-7 minutes of roasting. Keep an eye on them to avoid burning!

- Honey-glazed carrots make a great side dish for many plant-based meals.

Honey-glazed carrots are a sweet and nutritious side dish that combines the natural sweetness of carrots with the added benefits of honey. Carrots are a low-calorie, nutrient-dense food that is rich in vitamins, minerals, and antioxidants. Honey, on the other hand, contains antibacterial and antifungal properties, and is a natural sweetener that is rich in antioxidants.

Here are some of the key health benefits of honey-glazed carrots:

- Rich in Vitamins and Minerals: Carrots are a good source of vitamins A, K, potassium, and fiber.

- Antioxidant-Rich: Carrots contain antioxidants that help protect cells from damage.

- Supports Healthy Vision: The vitamin A in carrots supports healthy vision and can help prevent age-related macular degeneration.

- Supports Healthy Digestion: The fiber content in carrots can help promote healthy digestion and prevent constipation.

- Natural Sweetener: Honey is a natural sweetener that is rich in antioxidants and has antibacterial and antifungal properties.

- Nutritious and Delicious: Honey-glazed carrots are a tasty and nutritious side dish that can add flavor and nutrition to a variety of meals.

By incorporating honey-glazed carrots into your diet, you can enjoy a delicious and nutritious side dish that supports your overall health and well-being.

4. BALSAMIC GLAZED ASPARAGUS:

Drizzle asparagus spears with balsamic vinegar, olive oil, and minced garlic, then roast until tender and slightly charred for a flavorful and elegant side dish.
Here's a step-by-step guide on how to cook them:

Ingredients:
- 1 pound fresh asparagus spears, trimmed
- 2 tablespoons balsamic vinegar
- 1 tablespoon olive oil
- 2 cloves garlic, minced
- Salt and pepper, to taste

Instructions:
1. Preheat your oven to 425°F (220°C).
2. In a large bowl, whisk together balsamic vinegar, olive oil, and minced garlic.

3. Add the asparagus spears and toss to coat them evenly with the glaze.

4. Add salt and pepper to taste.

5. Spread the asparagus in a single layer on a baking sheet.

6. Roast in the preheated oven for 12-15 minutes, or until the asparagus is:

   - Tender: easily pierced with a fork

   - Slightly charred: caramelized and slightly browned on the outside

7. Remove from the oven and serve hot.

Tips:

- For optimal flavor, use premium balsamic vinegar.

-- Taste-test the garlic dosage.

- To enhance the caramelization process, increase the oven temperature to 450°F (230°C) for the last 2-3 minutes of roasting. Watch them to prevent burning!

- Balsamic glazed asparagus pairs well with many plant-based main dishes.

Balsamic glazed asparagus is a flavorful and nutritious vegetable dish that combines the natural goodness of asparagus with the rich flavor of balsamic glaze. Asparagus is a low-calorie, nutrient-dense food that is rich in vitamins, minerals, and antioxidants. Balsamic glaze, made from reduced balsamic vinegar, adds a sweet and tangy flavor without adding refined sugars.

Here are some of the key health benefits of balsamic glazed asparagus:

- Low in Calories: Asparagus is a low-calorie food that can help support weight management.

- Rich in Vitamins and Minerals: Asparagus is a good source of vitamins C and K, folate, and potassium.

- Antioxidant-Rich: Asparagus contains antioxidants that help protect cells from damage.

- Supports Healthy Digestion: The fiber content in asparagus can help promote healthy digestion and prevent constipation.

- May Help Lower Blood Pressure: The potassium content in asparagus can help lower blood pressure by counteracting the effects of sodium.

- Nutritious and Delicious: Balsamic glazed asparagus is a tasty and nutritious side dish that can add flavor and nutrition to a variety of meals.

By incorporating balsamic glazed asparagus into your diet, you can enjoy a delicious and nutritious vegetable dish that supports your overall health and well-being.

5. SAUTÉED SPINACH WITH GARLIC AND LEMON:

Cook fresh spinach with minced garlic, olive oil, and a squeeze of lemon juice until wilted and bright green for a vibrant and nutritious side.

Here's a simple recipe to make this vibrant and flavorful spinach:

Ingredients:
- 2 cups fresh spinach leaves
- 2 cloves garlic, minced
- 2 tablespoons olive oil
- 1 tablespoon lemon juice
- Add salt and pepper to taste.

Instructions:
1. Warm the olive oil in a large skillet over medium-low heat.
2. Add the minced garlic and sauté for 1-2 minutes until fragrant.
3. Add the fresh spinach leaves and sauté until wilted, about 2-3 minutes.
4. Squeeze the lemon juice over the spinach and season with salt and pepper to taste.
5. Serve hot and enjoy!

Tips:
- Use fresh and high-quality spinach for the best flavor.
- Taste-test the garlic quantity.

- For an intense kick, sprinkle it with red pepper flakes.
- Experiment with different citrus fruits, like lime or orange, for a unique flavor twist.

Sautéed spinach with garlic and lemon is a flavorful and nutritious vegetable dish that combines the natural goodness of spinach with the added benefits of garlic and lemon. Spinach is a low-calorie, nutrient-dense food that is rich in vitamins, minerals, and antioxidants. Garlic contains compounds that have antibacterial, antiviral, and antifungal properties, while lemon adds a burst of citrus flavor and a boost of vitamin C.
Here are some of the key health benefits of sautéed spinach with garlic and lemon:

- Rich in Vitamins and Minerals: Spinach is a good source of vitamins A, K, folate, and iron.

- Antioxidant-Rich: Spinach contains antioxidants that help protect cells from damage.
- Supports Healthy Eyesight: The vitamin A in spinach supports healthy vision and can help prevent age-related macular degeneration.

- Supports Healthy Bones: Spinach is a good source of calcium, which supports healthy bones.

- May Help Lower Blood Pressure: The potassium content in spinach can help lower blood pressure by counteracting the effects of sodium.

- Immune-Boosting Properties: Garlic contains compounds that have antibacterial, antiviral, and antifungal properties, which can help boost the immune system.

- Nutritious and Delicious: Sautéed spinach with garlic and lemon is a tasty and nutritious side dish that can add flavor and nutrition to a variety of meals.

By incorporating sautéed spinach with garlic and lemon into your diet, you can enjoy a delicious and nutritious vegetable dish that supports your overall health and well-being.

2.GRAIN AND LEGUME ACCOMPANIMENTS

1. QUINOA PILAF:

Cook quinoa with vegetable broth, diced onions, garlic, and your choice of herbs and spices until fluffy and fragrant for a nutritious and versatile side dish.
Here's a basic recipe you can customize with your favorite herbs and spices:

Ingredients:
- 1 cup quinoa, rinsed and drained
- 2 cups vegetable broth
- 1 small onion, diced
- 2 cloves garlic, minced
- 1 tablespoon olive oil
- Your choice of herbs and spices (e.g., paprika, cumin, coriander, thyme, rosemary)

Instructions:
In a small saucepan set over medium heat, warm the olive oil.
2. Cook, stirring, the diced onion until transparent, about 3–4 minutes.

3. Cook for a further minute after adding the minced garlic.

4. Add the quinoa and stir to coat with oil and mix with onion and garlic.

5. Add the veggie stock and heat through.

6. Reduce heat to low, cover, and simmer for about 15-20 minutes or until quinoa is fluffy and fragrant.

7. Fluff with a fork and season with your chosen herbs and spices.

Tips:

- For more taste, use vegetable broth rather than water.

- Customize with your favorite herbs and spices to match your main dish.

- Try adding other ingredients like diced bell peppers, chopped mushrooms, or toasted nuts for added texture and flavor.

- Quinoa pilaf is a great base for salads, bowls, or as a side dish on its own.

Quinoa pilaf is a nutritious and flavorful dish made with quinoa, a protein-rich grain that is native to the Andean region of South America. Quinoa is a complete protein, meaning that it includes all nine essential amino acids that the body cannot manufacture on its own.. It is also high in fiber, vitamins, and minerals, making it a nutritious and filling food.

Here are some of the key health benefits of quinoa pilaf:

- High in Protein: Quinoa is a complete protein, making it an excellent source of protein for vegetarians and vegans.

- Gluten-Free: Quinoa is gluten-free, making it a great option for people with gluten intolerance or celiac disease.

- Rich in Fiber: Quinoa is high in fiber, which can help lower cholesterol levels and promote healthy digestion.

- Antioxidant-Rich: Quinoa contains antioxidants like vitamin E and manganese, which can help protect cells from damage.

- May Help Lower Cholesterol: The fiber and protein in quinoa can help lower cholesterol levels and promote healthy heart function.

- Supports Healthy Blood Sugar Levels: Quinoa has a low glycemic index, making it a good choice for people with diabetes or those who want to manage their blood sugar levels.

- Nutritious and Delicious: Quinoa pilaf is a tasty and nutritious side dish that can add flavor and nutrition to a variety of meals.

By incorporating quinoa pilaf into your diet, you can enjoy a delicious and nutritious meal that supports your overall health and well-being.

2. LENTIL SALAD:

Toss cooked lentils with diced tomatoes, cucumbers, red onions, parsley, lemon juice, and olive oil for a refreshing and protein-packed side salad.

Here's a basic recipe you can customize to your taste:

Ingredients:
- 1 cup cooked lentils
- 1 cup diced tomatoes
- 1/2 cup diced cucumbers
- 1/4 cup diced red onions
- 1/4 cup chopped parsley
- 2 tablespoons lemon juice
- 1 tablespoon olive oil
- Salt and pepper to taste

Instructions:
1. In a large bowl, combine the cooked lentils, diced tomatoes, cucumbers, red onions, and parsley.
2. In a small bowl, mix together the lemon juice and olive oil.
3. Pour the dressing over the lentil mixture and toss to coat.

4. Season with salt and pepper to taste.

5. Serve chilled or at room temperature.

Tips:

- Use fresh and flavorful ingredients for the best taste.

- Customize the recipe with your preferred herbs and spices.

- Add other ingredients like diced bell peppers, chopped carrots, or crumbled feta cheese for added flavor and texture.

- Lentil salad is a great side dish for many meals, and it's also a good base for a light lunch or dinner.

Lentil salad is a nutritious and flavorful dish made with lentils, a type of legume that is rich in protein, fiber, and various vitamins and minerals. Lentils are a great source of plant-based protein and are low in calories, making them an excellent addition to a healthy diet.

Here are some of the key health benefits of lentil salad:

- High in protein: Vegans and vegetarians will find lentils to be a fantastic source of plant-based protein.

- Rich in Fiber: Lentils are high in fiber, which can help lower cholesterol levels, promote healthy digestion, and support healthy blood sugar levels.

- Low in Calories: Lentils are low in calories, making them an excellent addition to a weight loss diet.

- Antioxidant-Rich: Lentils contain antioxidants like polyphenols and flavonoids, which can help protect cells from damage.

- May Help Lower Cholesterol: The fiber and protein in lentils can help lower cholesterol levels and promote healthy heart function.

- Supports Healthy Blood Sugar Levels: Lentils have a low glycemic index, making them a good choice for people with diabetes or those who want to manage their blood sugar levels.

- Nutritious and Delicious: Lentil salad is a tasty and nutritious side dish that can add flavor and nutrition to a variety of meals.

By incorporating lentil salad into your diet, you can enjoy a delicious and nutritious meal that supports your overall health and well-being.

3. CHICKPEA CURRY:

Simmer cooked chickpeas with coconut milk, diced tomatoes, onions, garlic, ginger, and curry spices until thick and flavorful for a hearty and satisfying side dish. Here's a basic recipe you can customize to your taste:

Ingredients:
- 1 cup cooked chickpeas
- 1 cup coconut milk
- 1 cup diced tomatoes
- 1 small onion, diced
- 2 cloves garlic, minced
- 1-inch piece of ginger, grated
- 1 teaspoon curry powder
- 1 teaspoon ground cumin
- 1/2 teaspoon turmeric

- Salt and pepper, to taste

- Fresh cilantro, for garnish

Instructions:

1. In a large saucepan, sauté the onion, garlic, and ginger in a little oil until softened.

2. Add the curry powder, cumin, and turmeric and cook for 1-2 minutes, stirring constantly.

3. Stir in the coconut milk, diced tomatoes, and cooked chickpeas.

4. Bring to a simmer and cook until the sauce thickens, about 10-15 minutes.

5. To taste, add salt and pepper for seasoning.

6. Garnish with fresh cilantro and serve over rice or with naan bread.

Tips:

- Adjust the amount of curry spices to your desired level of heat.

- Add other ingredients like bell peppers, carrots, or potatoes for added flavor and texture.

- Use canned coconut milk for a creamy and rich sauce.

- Chickpea curry is a great side dish for many meals, and it's also a good base for a light lunch or dinner.

Chickpea curry is a flavorful and nutritious dish made with chickpeas, a type of legume that is rich in protein, fiber, and various vitamins and minerals. Chickpeas are a great source of plant-based protein and are low in calories, making them an excellent addition to a healthy diet. The curry sauce is typically made with a blend of spices, including turmeric, cumin, and coriander, which have anti-inflammatory and antioxidant properties.

Here are some of the key health benefits of chickpea curry:

- High in Protein: Chickpeas are a great source of plant-based protein, making them an excellent option for vegetarians and vegans.

- Rich in Fiber: Chickpeas are high in fiber, which can help lower cholesterol levels, promote healthy digestion, and support healthy blood sugar levels.

- Low in Calories: Chickpeas are low in calories, making them an excellent addition to a weight loss diet.

- Antioxidant-Rich: The spices in the curry sauce, such as turmeric and cumin, have anti-inflammatory and antioxidant properties.

- May Help Lower Cholesterol: The fiber and protein in chickpeas can help lower cholesterol levels and promote healthy heart function.

- Supports Healthy Blood Sugar Levels: Chickpeas have a low glycemic index, making them a good choice for people with diabetes or those who want to manage their blood sugar levels.

- Nutritious and Delicious: Chickpea curry is a tasty and nutritious meal that can add flavor and nutrition to a variety of meals.

By incorporating chickpea curry into your diet, you can enjoy a delicious and nutritious meal that supports your overall health and well-being.

4. BLACK BEAN AND CORN SALSA:

Combine black beans, corn kernels, diced tomatoes, red onions, cilantro, lime juice, and a dash of cumin for a colorful and flavorful plant-based side that pairs well with tacos or grilled portobello mushrooms.
To get you going, try this simple recipe:

Ingredients:
- 1 cup cooked black beans
- 1 cup corn kernels
- 1 cup diced tomatoes
- 1/2 cup diced red onion
- 1/4 cup chopped cilantro
- 2 tablespoons lime juice
- 1 teaspoon ground cumin
- Salt and pepper to taste

Instructions:
1. In a medium bowl, combine the black beans, corn kernels, diced tomatoes, red onion, and cilantro.
2. Squeeze the lime juice over the top and toss to coat.
3. Sprinkle the cumin over the mixture and season with salt and pepper to taste.

4. To let the flavors marry, cover and chill for at least half an hour.

5. Serve chilled or at room temperature alongside tacos, grilled portobello mushrooms, or as a dip for vegan chips.

Tips:

- Use fresh and flavorful ingredients for the best taste.
- Adjust the amount of lime juice and cumin to your liking.
- Add a diced jalapeño or serrano pepper for an extra kick of heat.
- This salsa is also great as a topping for vegan nachos or as a side dish for grilled vegetables. Enjoy!

Black bean and corn salsa is a delicious and nutritious condiment made with black beans, corn, and a blend of spices. This tasty topping is not only a great addition to your favorite dishes, but it's also packed with nutrients and antioxidants that can provide several health benefits.

Black beans are a great source of plant-based protein, fiber, and folate, making them an excellent option for vegetarians and vegans. They're also low in calories and rich in antioxidants, which can help protect against cell damage and reduce the risk of chronic diseases like heart disease and cancer.

Corn is a good source of vitamin C and thiamin, and it's also high in fiber and antioxidants. The fiber in corn can help promote healthy digestion and prevent constipation, while the antioxidants can help protect against cell damage and reduce inflammation.

When combined, black beans and corn create a powerful nutritional duo that's rich in protein, fiber, and antioxidants. The spices added to the salsa, such as cumin and chili powder, also have anti-inflammatory properties that can help reduce inflammation and improve overall health.

Some of the key health benefits of black bean and corn salsa include:

- High in protein and fiber, making it a great option for vegetarians and vegans
-Rich in antioxidants and low in calories, they can help guard against cell damage and lower the risk of chronic diseases.

- Might support a healthy digestive system and fend off constipation
- Possible to lower inflammation and enhance general health
- Can be used as a healthy topping for a variety of dishes, including salads, grilled meats, and vegetables

Black bean and corn salsa is a tasty and nutritious condiment that can add flavor and nutrition to a variety of meals.

5. BROWN RICE STIR-FRY:

Stir-fry cooked brown rice with mixed vegetables, tofu or tempeh, and a soy sauce-based sauce for a tasty and filling side dish that's easy to customize. It's a versatile and nutritious side dish that can be customized to suit your taste preferences. Here's a basic recipe to get you started:

Ingredients:
- Two cups of cooked brown rice, ideally from the previous day
- 1 cup mixed vegetables (e.g., broccoli, carrots, bell peppers, onions)
- 1/2 cup cubed tofu or tempeh
- 2 tablespoons soy sauce
- 1 tablespoon olive oil
- 1 teaspoon grated ginger
- 1 teaspoon garlic, minced
- Salt and pepper to taste
- Optional: other seasonings, herbs, or spices of your choice

Instructions:

1. To a large skillet or wok set over medium-high heat, add the olive oil.

2. Add the mixed vegetables and cook until they start to soften.

3. Add the cubed tofu or tempeh and cook until golden brown.

4. Add the cooked brown rice to the skillet or wok and stir-fry for about 5 minutes, breaking up any clumps with a spatula.

5. In a small bowl, whisk together the soy sauce, grated ginger, and garlic.

6. Pour the sauce over the rice mixture and stir-fry for another minute.

7. Season with salt, pepper, and any other desired herbs or spices.

8. Serve hot and enjoy!

Tips:

- Use leftover brown rice to make this dish.

- Customize with your favorite vegetables, herbs, and spices.

- Add protein sources like cooked chicken, shrimp, or edamame for added flavor and nutrition.

- Experiment with different sauces, such as hoisin sauce or sriracha, for a unique flavor profile.

Brown rice stir-fry is a popular and flavorful dish that combines the nutty taste of brown rice with the crunch and color of various vegetables, all tied together with a savory blend of spices. This tasty meal is a great way to get your daily dose of whole grains and veggies, making it a nutritious and satisfying option for a quick lunch or dinner.

Brown rice is a whole grain that's high in fiber and nutrients, including manganese, selenium, and magnesium. It's also a good source of protein and can help lower cholesterol levels and improve digestion. By using brown rice instead of white rice, you're getting a more nutritious and filling base for your meal.

The vegetables added to the stir-fry are rich in vitamins and minerals, and can vary depending on your personal preferences and dietary needs. Some common vegetables used in brown rice stir-fry include broccoli, bell peppers, carrots, and snap peas. These veggies add crunch, flavor, and texture to the dish, making it a well-rounded and satisfying meal.

The blend of spices used in brown rice stir-fry can also vary, but common ingredients include soy sauce, garlic, ginger, and chili flakes. These spices add depth and flavor to the dish, and can be adjusted to suit your personal taste preferences.

Brown rice stir-fry is a tasty and nutritious meal that's easy to make and customize to your liking. It's a great option for a quick and easy meal that's packed with whole grains, veggies, and flavor.

3. EASY-TO-MAKE SIDE SALADS

1. CLASSIC CAPRESE SALAD:

Arrange sliced tomatoes, fresh mozzarella cheese, and basil leaves on a platter, then drizzle with balsamic glaze and olive oil for a simple yet elegant side salad.

The Classic Caprese Salad is a timeless and flavorful Italian dish that showcases the simplicity and elegance of fresh ingredients. This iconic salad is composed of three main components: juicy tomatoes, creamy mozzarella cheese, and fragrant basil leaves, dressed with extra virgin olive oil and a sprinkle of salt.

The tomatoes used in the Caprese Salad are typically ripe and flavorful, providing a sweet and tangy base for the dish. The mozzarella cheese adds a rich and creamy element, while the fresh basil leaves provide a bright and herbaceous note. The extra virgin olive oil brings everything together, adding a smooth and velvety texture to the salad.

This salad is a celebration of the flavors and ingredients of Italy, and is often served as an antipasto or side dish. It's a great way to experience the freshness and quality of the ingredients, and is perfect for warm weather or outdoor gatherings.

Some of the key ingredients in the Classic Caprese Salad include:

- Fresh tomatoes
- Mozzarella cheese
- Fresh basil leaves
- Extra virgin olive oil
- Salt

This salad is a great option for those looking for a light and refreshing meal that's packed with flavor and freshness. It's also a great way to support local farmers and artisanal producers, as the ingredients can be sourced from local markets and farms.

2. CUCUMBER TOMATO SALAD:

Toss sliced cucumbers and cherry tomatoes with red onions, feta cheese, olives, and a Greek vinaigrette dressing for a refreshing and flavorful side dish.

Cucumber Tomato Salad is a nutritious and refreshing dish that offers numerous health benefits due to its high content of vitamins, minerals, and antioxidants.

1. Hydration: Cucumbers are made up of about 96% water, making them an excellent source of hydration.

2. Antioxidant properties: Tomatoes are rich in lycopene, an antioxidant that helps protect cells from damage and reduces the risk of certain cancers.

3. Anti-inflammatory effects: Cucumbers contain anti-inflammatory compounds like fisetin, which may help reduce inflammation and improve overall health.

4. Digestive health: Cucumbers contain fiber and water, making them beneficial for digestive health and promoting regular bowel movements.

5. Vitamin and mineral boost: Tomatoes are a good source of vitamins A and C, potassium, and folate, while cucumbers provide vitamin K and potassium.

6. Low calorie count: This salad is very low in calories, making it an excellent addition to a weight management diet.

7. Anti-cancer properties: The antioxidants and other compounds in tomatoes and cucumbers may help reduce the risk of certain cancers, such as prostate, breast, and colon cancer.

8. Cardiovascular health: The potassium content in both tomatoes and cucumbers can help lower blood pressure and support overall cardiovascular health.

Enjoy your Cucumber Tomato Salad, knowing it's not only delicious but also packed with nutrients and health benefits.

3. KALE CAESAR SALAD:

 Massage chopped kale leaves with Caesar dressing until tender, then toss with croutons, shaved Parmesan cheese, and freshly ground black pepper for a modern twist on a classic salad.

Kale Caesar Salad is a nutritious and delicious twist on the classic Caesar Salad. By substituting kale for traditional lettuce, this salad packs a powerful punch of vitamins, minerals, and antioxidants.

The Following are some of the main health benefits:

1. High in Vitamins: Kale is rich in vitamins A, C, and K, as well as minerals like calcium and iron.

2. Antioxidant Properties: Kale contains a high amount of antioxidants, which help protect cells from damage and reduce the risk of chronic diseases.

3. Anti-Inflammatory Effects: Kale contains compounds like isothiocyanates, which may help reduce inflammation and improve overall health.

4. Supports Eye Health: The high levels of lutein and zeaxanthin in kale make it an excellent food for supporting eye health and reducing the risk of age-related macular degeneration.

5. May Support Detoxification: Kale contains compounds that may help support the body's natural detoxification processes.

6. High in Fiber: Kale is high in fiber, which can help promote digestive health and support healthy blood sugar levels.

7. Supports Bone Health: Kale is a good source of calcium, which is essential for maintaining strong bones.

8. May Support Heart Health: The potassium content in kale can help lower blood pressure and support overall cardiovascular health.

By combining kale with the other ingredients in a Caesar Salad, like protein-rich chickpeas and healthy fats from olive oil, you create a salad that is both delicious and nutritious.

4. BEET AND GOAT CHEESE SALAD:

Roast or steam beets until tender, then slice and toss with mixed greens, crumbled goat cheese, toasted walnuts, and a balsamic vinaigrette for a colorful and elegant side salad.

Beet and Goat Cheese Salad is a delicious and nutritious combination of flavors and textures. Beets are a rich source of vitamins, minerals, and antioxidants, while goat cheese provides a boost of protein and calcium.

The Following are some of the main health benefits:

1. Antioxidant Properties: Beets contain a unique antioxidant called betalain, which has anti-inflammatory properties and may help reduce the risk of chronic diseases.

2. Supports Heart Health: The fiber, potassium, and antioxidants in beets may help lower blood pressure and support overall cardiovascular health.

117

3. May Support Detoxification: Beets contain compounds that may help support the body's natural detoxification processes.

4. High in Fiber: Beets are high in fiber, which can help promote digestive health and support healthy blood sugar levels.

5. Good Source of Vitamins and Minerals: Beets are a good source of vitamins A, C, and K, as well as minerals like potassium, magnesium, and iron.

6. Protein-Rich Goat Cheese: Goat cheese provides a boost of protein, which can help support muscle health and satisfaction.

7. Supports Bone Health: Goat cheese is a good source of calcium, which is essential for maintaining strong bones.

8. May Support Immune Function: The probiotics in goat cheese may help support immune function and promote a healthy gut microbiome.

Enjoy your Beet and Goat Cheese Salad, knowing it's not only delicious but also packed with nutrients and health benefits.

5. QUINOA TABOULI SALAD:

Combine cooked quinoa with chopped tomatoes, cucumbers, red onions, parsley, mint, lemon juice, and olive oil for a refreshing and nutritious side salad with a Mediterranean flair.

Quinoa Tabouli Salad is a nutritious and refreshing twist on the classic Middle Eastern dish. By using quinoa instead of bulgur, this salad packs a protein and fiber punch.

The Following are some of the main health benefits:

1. Complete Protein: Quinoa is a complete protein, meaning it contains all nine essential amino acids that the body can't produce on its own.

2. High in Fiber: Quinoa is high in fiber, which can help promote digestive health and support healthy blood sugar levels.

3. Gluten-Free: Quinoa is gluten-free, making it an excellent option for those with gluten intolerance or sensitivity.

4. Antioxidant Properties: The herbs and vegetables in tabouli, such as parsley, tomatoes, and mint, contain antioxidants that help protect cells from damage.

5. Supports Heart Health: The fiber, potassium, and antioxidants in quinoa and tabouli may help lower blood pressure and support overall cardiovascular health.
6. May Support Detoxification: The parsley and lemon juice in tabouli may help support the body's natural detoxification processes.
7. Good Source of Vitamins and Minerals: Quinoa and tabouli are good sources of vitamins A, C, and K, as well as minerals like iron, magnesium, and potassium.
8. Supports Healthy Gut Bacteria: The fiber in quinoa can help feed good gut bacteria, promoting a healthy gut microbiome.

Enjoy your Quinoa Tabouli Salad, knowing it's not only delicious but also packed with nutrients and health benefits.

CHAPTER 6

DESSERTS TO SATISFY

1. DECADENT PLANT-BASED DESSERT RECIPES

1. VEGAN CHOCOLATE AVOCADO MOUSSE:

Blend ripe avocados with cocoa powder, maple syrup, and vanilla extract until smooth and creamy for a rich and indulgent chocolate mousse.

Vegan chocolate avocado mousse is a decadent and delicious dessert! Here's a simple recipe to make this rich and creamy treat:

Ingredients:
- 3 ripe avocados
- 1/2 cup cocoa powder
- 1/4 cup maple syrup

- 1 teaspoon vanilla extract

- Pinch of salt

Instructions:

1. Put the avocados, pitted and peeled, into a food processor or blender.

2. Add the cocoa powder, maple syrup, vanilla extract, and salt to the blender.

3. Blend the mixture on high speed until smooth and creamy, stopping to scrape down the sides of the blender as needed.

4. Pour the mousse into individual serving cups or a large serving dish.

5. Serve cold, having chilled for at least two hours in the refrigerator.

6. Garnish with fresh fruit, nuts, or shaved chocolate, if desired.

Tips:

- Use ripe avocados for the best creamy texture.

- Taste-test the maple syrup to see how sweet you want it.

- Add a pinch of cinnamon or nutmeg for extra depth of flavor.

- Experiment with different types of non-dairy milk or flavorings, like coconut milk or orange extract, for unique variations.

Enjoy your rich and indulgent vegan chocolate avocado mousse!

Vegan Chocolate Avocado Mousse is a rich and creamy dessert that's not only delicious but also packed with nutrients. Avocados provide healthy fats, while cocoa powder and maple syrup offer a boost of antioxidants and flavonoids.

Several main health benefits are as follows:

1. Healthy Fats: Avocados contain monounsaturated fats that support heart health and satisfy hunger.

2. Antioxidant Properties: Cocoa powder and maple syrup contain antioxidants that help protect cells from damage and reduce inflammation.

3. May Improve Heart Health: The flavonoids in cocoa powder may help lower blood pressure and improve blood flow.

4. Supports Healthy Bones: Avocados contain vitamin K, which supports bone health and density.

5. Good Source of Fiber: Avocados are high in fiber, which promotes digestive health and supports healthy blood sugar levels.

6. May Improve Mood: The tryptophan in avocados and the phenylethylamine in chocolate may help boost mood and reduce stress.

7. Supports Healthy Skin: The healthy fats in avocados and antioxidants in cocoa powder may help nourish and protect the skin.

8. Vegan and Dairy-Free: This dessert is perfect for those with dairy allergies or intolerances, or those following a vegan lifestyle.

Enjoy your Vegan Chocolate Avocado Mousse, knowing it's not only decadent but also nutritious.

2. DAIRY-FREE COCONUT MILK ICE CREAM:

Mix full-fat coconut milk with sweetener and vanilla extract, then churn in an ice cream maker until creamy and frozen for a refreshing and dairy-free dessert. Dairy-free coconut milk ice cream is a delicious and refreshing dessert option! Here's a basic recipe to get you started:

Ingredients:
- 1 can full-fat coconut milk
- 1/4 cup sweetener (e.g., maple syrup, coconut sugar, or dates)
- 1 teaspoon vanilla extract

Instructions:
1. Open the coconut milk can and scoop out the solid coconut cream into a blender or food processor.
2. Add the sweetener and vanilla extract to the blender.
3. Process the blend until it's creamy and smooth.
4. Transfer the blend into an ice cream maker and process in accordance with the guidelines provided by the manufacturer.

5. Once churned, transfer the ice cream to an airtight container and freeze for at least 2 hours to firm up.
6. Enjoy your dairy-free coconut milk ice cream!

Tips:
- Coconut milk with full fat will have the creamiest texture.
- Adjust the sweetener to your taste preferences.
- Add mix-ins like cocoa powder, nuts, or fruit to create different flavors.
- If you don't have an ice cream maker, you can also freeze the mixture in a container and blend it every 30 minutes until the desired consistency is reached.

Dairy-Free Coconut Milk Ice Cream is a delicious and refreshing dessert option that's perfect for those with dairy allergies or intolerances. Coconut milk provides a creamy texture and a boost of nutrients.

1. Dairy-Free: Perfect for those with dairy allergies or intolerances.

2. Rich in Medium-Chain Triglycerides (MCTs): Coconut milk contains MCTs, which are easily absorbed and can provide a quick source of energy.

3. Supports Immune System: Coconut milk contains lauric acid, a compound with antimicrobial and antifungal properties that can help support the immune system.

4. May Support Weight Loss: The MCTs in coconut milk may help increase satiety and boost metabolism.

5. Good Source of Fiber: Coconut milk contains fiber, which can help promote digestive health.

6. May Support Healthy Cholesterol Levels: The medium-chain fatty acids in coconut milk may help raise HDL (good) cholesterol levels.

7. Supports Healthy Skin: The antioxidants and fatty acids in coconut milk may help nourish and protect the skin.

8. Vegan and Plant-Based: Perfect for those following a plant-based diet.

Enjoy your Dairy-Free Coconut Milk Ice Cream, knowing it's not only delicious but also nutritious.

3. ALMOND FLOUR CHOCOLATE CHIP COOKIES:

Combine almond flour, coconut oil, maple syrup, and chocolate chips to make soft and chewy chocolate chip cookies that are gluten-free and delicious.
Almond flour chocolate chip cookies are a delicious and gluten-free treat. Here's a simple recipe to make these soft and chewy cookies:

Ingredients:
- 1 1/2 cups almond flour
- 1/4 cup coconut oil
- 1/4 cup maple syrup
- 1/2 cup chocolate chips
- 2 eggs
- 1 teaspoon vanilla extract
- Pinch of salt

Instructions:
- Preheat the oven to 350°F (175°C). Line a baking sheet with parchment paper.
- In a large bowl, combine almond flour, coconut oil, maple syrup, and mix until well combined.

- Add eggs, vanilla extract, and salt. Mix until a dough forms.

- Fold in chocolate chips.

- Using a tablespoon-sized scoop, place dough balls onto the baking sheet that has been prepared, allowing 2 inches between each cookie.

- Bake for 10-11 minutes or until lightly golden brown.

- Take out of the oven and allow to cool for five minutes on the baking sheet, then move to a wire rack to cool down completely.

Tips:

- Use fine almond flour for the best results.

- Coconut oil can be replaced with butter or other dairy-free alternatives.

- Add nuts or dried fruit to change up the flavor.

- Cookies can be frozen for up to three months or kept for up to five days at room temperature in an airtight container.

Almond Flour Chocolate Chip Cookies are a nutritious and delicious treat that offers several health benefits. With almond flour, these cookies are:

1. Gluten-free, perfect for those with gluten intolerance or sensitivity.

2. High in protein, supporting muscle health and satisfaction.

3. Rich in healthy fats, lowering cholesterol levels and regulating blood sugar levels.

4. A good source of fiber, promoting digestive health and satiety.

5. Supportive of healthy bones, with calcium, magnesium, and phosphorus.

6. Lower in carbohydrates, making them a great option for low-carb diets.

7. Made with minimal ingredients, reducing the risk of allergic reactions and intolerances.

8. Delicious and satisfying, making them a great treat for any time of day.

Enjoy your Almond Flour Chocolate Chip Cookies, knowing they're a healthy and delicious choice.

4. RAW VEGAN CHEESECAKE:

Blend cashews, coconut cream, dates, and lemon juice until smooth, then pour over a nut and date crust and chill until set for a creamy and luscious raw vegan cheesecake.

Raw vegan cheesecake is a delicious and creamy dessert option! Here's a basic recipe to make this luscious treat:

Ingredients:

For the crust:
- 1 cup nuts (e.g., almonds or walnuts)
- 1 cup dates
- 1/4 cup coconut oil

134

For the filling:

- 1 1/2 cups cashews

- 1 cup coconut cream

- 1/2 cup dates

- 2 tablespoons lemon juice

- 1/4 teaspoon salt

- 1/2 teaspoon vanilla extract

Instructions:

1. Soak the cashews in water for at least 4 hours or overnight.

2. Drain and rinse the cashews, then add them to a blender with the remaining filling ingredients.

3. Blend until smooth and creamy, stopping to scrape down the sides of the blender as needed.

4. Pour the filling over the prepared crust and chill in the refrigerator for at least 4 hours or until set.

5. Enjoy your raw vegan cheesecake!

Tips:

- Use a high-speed blender like Vitamix or Blendtec for the smoothest texture.

- Adjust the sweetness and flavor to your liking by adding more dates or lemon juice.
- For extra taste and texture, sprinkle nuts or fresh fruit on top.
- Experiment with different flavors like cocoa powder or matcha powder for a unique twist.

Raw Vegan Cheesecake is a delicious and nutritious dessert option that's perfect for those following a plant-based diet. Made with cashews, coconut cream, and natural sweeteners, this cheesecake offers several health benefits:

1. Dairy-free and cruelty-free, making it a great option for those with dairy allergies or intolerances.

2. High in healthy fats from cashews and coconut cream, supporting heart health and satiety.

3. Rich in antioxidants and vitamins from fresh fruit and natural sweeteners.

4. Good source of fiber and protein from cashews and coconut.

5. Supports healthy digestion with probiotics from fermented cashews.

6. May help lower cholesterol levels with plant sterols from cashews.

7. No refined sugars or artificial ingredients, making it a great option for those looking for a healthier dessert.

8. Supports healthy weight management with nutrient-dense ingredients.

Enjoy your Raw Vegan Cheesecake, knowing it's a delicious and nutritious treat.

5. PEANUT BUTTER BANANA ICE CREAM:

Blend frozen bananas with peanut butter and a splash of almond milk until creamy, then freeze until firm for a guilt-free and delicious banana ice cream.
Peanut butter banana ice cream is a delicious and guilt-free treat! Here's a simple recipe to make this creamy and dreamy ice cream:

Ingredients:

- 3-4 frozen bananas
- 2 tablespoons peanut butter
- 1/4 cup almond milk
- Pinch of salt

Instructions:

1. Add the frozen bananas, peanut butter, almond milk, and salt to a blender.
2. Blend the mixture on high speed until smooth and creamy, stopping to scrape down the sides of the blender as needed.
3. Pour the mixture into a container and freeze for at least 2 hours or until firm.

4. Scoop and enjoy!

Tips:

- Use ripe bananas for the best flavor.
- Adjust the amount of peanut butter to your taste.
- Add other ingredients like cocoa powder, honey, or chopped nuts to change up the flavor.
- Experiment with different non-dairy milks like coconut milk or cashew milk for a creamier texture.

Peanut Butter Banana Ice Cream is a nutritious and delicious dessert that offers numerous health benefits. Made with frozen bananas, peanut butter, and natural sweeteners, this ice cream is:

1. Dairy-free, perfect for those with dairy allergies or intolerances.

2. Rich in potassium, supporting healthy blood pressure, muscle function, and heart health.

3. A good source of healthy fats, supporting heart health, satiety, and weight management.

4. High in fiber, promoting digestive health, satiety, and blood sugar control.

5. A good source of protein, supporting muscle health, satisfaction, and weight management.

6. Free from refined sugars and artificial ingredients, making it a healthier dessert option.

7. Supports healthy weight management with nutrient-dense ingredients.

8. Can help satisfy sweet cravings without compromising nutrition.
9. May help reduce inflammation with antioxidants from peanut butter and bananas.

10. Supports healthy bones with potassium, magnesium, and other minerals.

Enjoy your Peanut Butter Banana Ice Cream, knowing it's a healthy, delicious, and nutritious treat.

2. HEALTHY TREATS FOR SWEET CRAVINGS

1. FROZEN GRAPES:

Freeze fresh grapes until firm for a refreshing and naturally sweet frozen treat that's perfect for satisfying sweet cravings.

Frozen Grapes are a sweet and nutritious snack that offers several health benefits. These frozen treats are:

1. High in Vitamins C and K, which promote bone health and immune system.
2. High in Antioxidants, protecting cells from damage and reducing inflammation.
3. Good source of Potassium, supporting healthy blood pressure and heart function.
4. Low in Calories, making them a great snack for weight management.
5. Free from Added Sugars, making them a healthier option compared to other frozen treats.
6. Support Healthy Digestion with fiber and water content.
7. May Help Reduce Inflammation and Improve Heart Health with resveratrol.

8. Can Help Support Healthy Bones with calcium and other minerals.

9. Versatile and Convenient, perfect for snacking on the go!

10. A Healthy Alternative to traditional frozen treats like ice cream or popsicles.

Enjoy your Frozen Grapes, knowing they're a delicious and nutritious choice!

2. APPLE NACHOS:

 Slice apples into rounds and arrange on a plate, then drizzle with almond butter, honey, and sprinkle with granola, nuts, and chocolate chips for a fun and nutritious snack.

Apple Nachos are a delicious and nutritious snack made with fresh apples, nut butter, and optional toppings like cinnamon or oats. Unlike traditional nachos, Apple Nachos are a healthier alternative that offers numerous health benefits without compromising on taste.

Here are the health benefits of Apple Nachos:

- High in Fiber: Apples are a rich source of dietary fiber, which can help regulate bowel movements, prevent constipation, and support healthy digestion.

- Antioxidant-Rich: Apples contain a range of antioxidants, including vitamin C and polyphenols, which can help protect cells from damage, reduce inflammation, and support overall health.

- Healthy Fats: Nut butters like peanut butter or almond butter provide healthy fats that support heart health, regulate blood sugar levels, and improve insulin sensitivity.

- Supports Healthy Bones: Apples are a good source of boron, a mineral that is essential for maintaining healthy bones and preventing osteoporosis.

- May Help Reduce Cancer Risk: The antioxidants and phytonutrients in apples have been shown to have anti-cancer properties, and may help reduce the risk of certain types of cancer.

- Supports Healthy Immune Function: Apples contain a range of immune-boosting compounds, including vitamin C and polyphenols, which can help support healthy immune function and reduce the risk of illness.

Remember, Apple Nachos are a healthier snack option that can be enjoyed in moderation as part of a balanced diet. Savor your tasty and nourishing Apple Nachos.

3. GREEK YOGURT PARFAIT:

Layer Greek yogurt with sliced fruits, nuts, seeds, and a drizzle of honey for a protein-packed and satisfying dessert or snack.

Greek Yogurt Parfait is a nutritious and delicious snack or dessert made with Greek yogurt, granola, and fresh fruits.

Here are the health benefits of Greek Yogurt Parfait:

- High in Protein: Greek yogurt is an excellent source of protein, which can help build and repair muscles, support weight management, and regulate appetite.

- Good Source of Calcium: Greek yogurt is rich in calcium, essential for building and maintaining strong bones and teeth, and supporting muscle function.

- Probiotics: Greek yogurt contains live and active cultures, which can help support healthy digestion, boost the immune system, and regulate bowel movements.

- Fiber-Rich: Granola and fruits in the parfait provide fiber, which can help regulate bowel movements, prevent constipation, and support healthy digestion.

- Antioxidant-Rich: Fresh fruits in the parfait are rich in antioxidants, which can help protect cells from damage, reduce inflammation, and support overall health.

- Supports Healthy Blood Sugar Levels: Greek yogurt and fruits in the parfait can help regulate blood sugar levels and improve insulin sensitivity.

- Supports Healthy Weight Management: Greek yogurt and fiber-rich granola and fruits can help regulate appetite, support healthy weight management, and reduce the risk of chronic diseases.
Enjoy your Greek Yogurt Parfait, a delicious and nutritious treat.

4. CHOCOLATE COVERED STRAWBERRIES:

Dip fresh strawberries in melted dark chocolate, then place on a parchment-lined tray and refrigerate until the chocolate sets for a simple and elegant sweet treat.

In the realm of sweet indulgences, few treats rival the allure of chocolate-covered strawberries. This match made in heaven not only tantalizes the taste buds but also bestows a plethora of health benefits upon those who partake in its delightful union.

- Strawberry Bliss: Fresh strawberries burst with vitamin C, a potent antioxidant that shields the body from oxidative stress and inflammation, fostering a radiant glow from the inside out.

- Chocolate Charm: Dark chocolate's flavonoids and polyphenols join forces to improve blood flow, boost cognitive function, and even lower blood pressure, making this sweet treat a heart-healthy delight.

- Fruitful Fusion: The synergy of strawberry and chocolate creates a powerful anti-inflammatory effect, bolstering the immune system and protecting against chronic diseases.

- Sweet Serenade: Indulging in chocolate-covered strawberries releases endorphins, bathing the brain in a warm embrace of happiness and relaxation, making this treat a sweet escape from the stresses of everyday life.

- Berry Beautiful Skin: The vitamin C and alpha-hydroxy acid in strawberries work in harmony to brighten and smooth the skin, revealing a radiant complexion that glows with health and vitality.

- Chocolate's Gift: Dark chocolate's flavonoids improve blood flow to the skin, enhancing its natural glow and leaving you with a luscious, healthy complexion that's simply irresistible.

In the world of chocolate-covered strawberries, indulgence meets nutrition, and the result is a treat that's as delicious as it is nutritious. So go ahead, indulge in this sweet delight, and let the health benefits be your sweet reward!

5. CHIA SEED PUDDING:

Mix chia seeds with your choice of milk and sweetener, then let sit in the refrigerator until thickened for a creamy and nutritious pudding that's perfect for satisfying sweet cravings.

Chia seed pudding is a delicious and healthy dessert made by soaking chia seeds in liquid, typically almond milk or coconut milk, and sweetening it with natural sweeteners like honey or maple syrup. This tasty treat is not only delicious but also packed with nutrients and health benefits.

- Omega-3 Rich: Chia seeds are an excellent source of alpha-linolenic acid (ALA), a type of omega-3 fatty acid that supports heart health by reducing inflammation and improving blood lipid profiles.

- High in Fiber: Chia seeds are packed with dietary fiber, containing both soluble and insoluble fiber. This high fiber content supports healthy digestion, promotes satiety, and helps regulate blood sugar levels.

- Complete Protein Source: Chia seeds contain all nine essential amino acids, making them a complete protein source that supports muscle growth and repair.

- Antioxidant Powerhouse: Chia seeds contain a rich array of antioxidants, including chlorogenic acid, caffeic acid, and quercetin, which protect the body from oxidative stress and inflammation, reducing the risk of chronic diseases.

- Hydrating Properties: Chia seeds have the ability to absorb up to 10 times their weight in water, making them an excellent source of hydration and supporting healthy fluid balance in the body.

- Gluten-Free: Chia seeds are naturally gluten-free, making them a great option for those with gluten intolerance or sensitivity.
- Low in Calories: Chia seed pudding is relatively low in calories, making it a guilt-free treat that won't compromise your dietary goals.

By incorporating chia seed pudding into your diet, you can reap these nutritional benefits and support your overall health and well-being.

3. FRUIT-FOCUSED DELIGHTS

1. GRILLED PINEAPPLE WITH CINNAMON:

Grill pineapple slices until caramelized and fragrant, then sprinkle with cinnamon and serve for a simple and delicious dessert or snack.

Here's a simple recipe to make this sweet and flavorful treat:

Ingredients:

- 1 ripe pineapple, sliced into 1-inch rings
- 1/4 teaspoon ground cinnamon
- 1 tablespoon brown sugar (optional)

Instructions:

1. Preheat your grill to medium heat.
2. In a small bowl, mix together cinnamon and brown sugar (if using).
3. Brush both sides of the pineapple slices with the cinnamon-sugar mixture.
4. Grill the pineapple slices for 2-3 minutes per side, or until caramelized and fragrant.
5. Serve warm and enjoy!

Tips:

- For optimal results, use a pineapple that is firm yet ripe.
- To suit your taste, vary the amount of sugar and cinnamon.
- Add a splash of rum or vanilla extract for extra flavor.
- Grill pineapple slices on a skewer with other fruits, like peaches or bananas, for a colorful and tasty kebab.

Grilled Pineapple with Cinnamon is a delicious and nutritious dessert or snack that offers several health benefits.

Here are some of the benefits:

- Antioxidant-Rich: Pineapple is a rich source of antioxidants, including vitamin C and beta-carotene, which help protect cells from damage, reduce inflammation, and support overall health.

- Anti-Inflammatory Effects: Pineapple contains anti-inflammatory compounds like bromelain, which can help reduce inflammation and improve symptoms of conditions like arthritis, gout, and sinusitis.

- Supports Healthy Digestion: Pineapple is a good source
of dietary fiber, which can help regulate bowel
movements, prevent constipation, and support healthy
digestion.

- May Help Reduce Cancer Risk: The antioxidants and
phytonutrients in pineapple have been shown to have
anti-cancer properties, and may help reduce the risk of
certain types of cancer.

- Supports Healthy Bones: Pineapple is a good source of
manganese, a mineral that is essential for bone health
and may help prevent osteoporosis.

- Cinnamon Adds Extra Benefits: Cinnamon has
anti-inflammatory properties, can help regulate blood
sugar levels, and may improve heart health.

- Low in Calories: Grilled pineapple with cinnamon is a
low-calorie dessert or snack option, making it a great
choice for those watching their weight.

Enjoy your grilled pineapple with cinnamon, a delicious
and nutritious treat.

2. BERRY SALAD WITH MINT:

Toss mixed berries with fresh mint leaves, lemon zest, and a drizzle of honey or maple syrup for a refreshing and light fruit salad that's bursting with flavor. Here's a simple recipe to make this sweet and tangy treat:

Ingredients:

- Two cups of mixed berries, including blackberries, raspberries, blueberries, and strawberries
- 1/4 cup fresh mint leaves, chopped
- 1 tablespoon lemon zest
- 2 tablespoons honey or maple syrup

Instructions:

1. In a large bowl, combine the mixed berries and chopped mint leaves.
2. In a small bowl, whisk together lemon zest and honey or maple syrup until well combined.
3. Pour the lemon-honey dressing over the berry mixture and toss to coat.
4. Serve immediately and enjoy!

Tips:

- Use fresh and flavorful berries for the best taste.

- To taste, adjust the amount of mint.

- Add a splash of lemon juice for extra tartness.

- Substitute other herbs like basil or lemongrass for a unique flavor twist.

Berry Salad with Mint is a refreshing and nutritious dessert or snack that offers numerous health benefits.

Here are some of the benefits:

- Antioxidant-Rich: Berries are packed with antioxidants, including anthocyanins, ellagic acid, and quercetin, which help protect cells from damage, reduce inflammation, and support overall health.

- May Help Reduce Heart Disease Risk: The antioxidants and fiber in berries may help lower cholesterol levels, blood pressure, and inflammation, reducing the risk of heart disease.

- Supports Healthy Brain Function: Berries contain compounds that may help improve memory, cognitive function, and mood.

- May Help Manage Blood Sugar Levels: Berries are low in sugar and high in fiber, making them a good choice for those with diabetes or trying to manage blood sugar levels.

- Supports Healthy Digestion: Berries are a good source of dietary fiber, which can help regulate bowel movements, prevent constipation, and support healthy digestion.

- Mint Adds Extra Benefits: Mint may help improve digestion, reduce nausea and headaches, and support healthy immune function.

- Low in Calories: Berry salad with mint is a low-calorie dessert or snack option, making it a great choice for those watching their weight.

- Supports Healthy Bones: Berries are a good source of manganese, vitamin K, and calcium, which are essential for bone health.

Enjoy your berry salad with mint, a delicious and nutritious treat.

3. MANGO COCONUT RICE PUDDING:

Cook rice with coconut milk, diced mangoes, and a touch of sweetener until creamy and tender for a tropical-inspired rice pudding that's perfect for dessert or breakfast.

Here's a simple recipe to make this creamy and flavorful pudding:

Ingredients:
- One cup of raw brown or white rice
- 2 cups coconut milk
- 1 cup diced fresh mango
- 2 tablespoons sweetener (e.g., sugar, honey, or maple syrup)
- Pinch of salt
- Optional: 1/4 teaspoon ground cinnamon or nutmeg

Instructions:

1. Rinse the rice and combine with coconut milk, mango, sweetener, and salt in a medium saucepan.
2. Cook over medium heat, stirring constantly, until the rice is tender and the mixture is creamy.
3. Reduce heat to low and simmer for 5-7 minutes or until the pudding has thickened.
4. Stir in cinnamon or nutmeg, if using.
5. Serve warm or chilled, garnished with additional mango slices and toasted coconut flakes, if desired.

Tips:

- Use fresh and ripe mango for the best flavor.
- Adjust the amount of sweetener to your taste.
- Add a splash of lime juice for extra brightness.
- Experiment with different spices, like cardamom or ginger, for unique flavor twists.

Mango Coconut Rice Pudding is a delicious and nutritious dessert that offers several health benefits.

Here are some of the benefits:

- Rich in Fiber: Rice pudding is a good source of fiber, which can help regulate bowel movements, prevent constipation, and support healthy digestion.

- Antioxidant-Rich: Mango is packed with antioxidants, including vitamin C and beta-carotene, which help protect cells from damage, reduce inflammation, and support overall health.
- Healthy Fats: Coconut milk contains healthy fats that support heart health, regulate blood sugar levels, and improve digestion.

- May Help Lower Cholesterol: The fiber and healthy fats in Mango Coconut Rice Pudding may help lower cholesterol levels and improve blood lipid profiles.

- Supports Healthy Bones: Mango is a good source of vitamin K and potassium, which are essential for bone health.

- Can Help Manage Blood Sugar Levels: The fiber and healthy fats in Mango Coconut Rice Pudding may help regulate blood sugar levels and improve insulin sensitivity.

- Supports Healthy Gut Bacteria: The prebiotic fiber in rice pudding can help feed good gut bacteria, supporting a healthy gut microbiome.
- May Help Reduce Inflammation: The antioxidants and anti-inflammatory compounds in Mango Coconut Rice Pudding may help reduce inflammation and improve overall health.
Enjoy your Mango Coconut Rice Pudding, a delicious and nutritious treat.

4. WATERMELON SORBET:

Puree fresh watermelon chunks until smooth, then freeze in an ice cream maker until firm for a refreshing and naturally sweet sorbet that's perfect for hot summer days. Watermelon sorbet is a refreshing and delicious dessert perfect for hot summer days! Here's a simple recipe to make this naturally sweet and refreshing sorbet:

Ingredients:

- 3-4 cups fresh watermelon chunks (seedless)
- 1 tablespoon lime juice (optional)

Instructions:

1. In a blender or food processor, puree the watermelon chunks until smooth.
2. Strain the mixture through a fine-mesh sieve to remove any excess pulp or fibers.
3. Add lime juice, if using, and stir to combine.
4. Transfer the blend into an ice cream maker and process in accordance with the guidelines provided by the manufacturer.
5. Once frozen and firm, scoop and enjoy!

Tips:

- For the greatest taste, use sweet, ripe watermelon.
- Tailor the lime juice to your personal preference.
- For a cool twist, add a dash of sparkling water.
- Experiment with different flavors, like mint or basil, for unique variations.
Watermelon Sorbet is a refreshing and nutritious dessert that offers several health benefits.

Here are some of the benefits:
- Hydrating: Watermelon is made up of about 92% water, making it an excellent source of hydration.

- Antioxidant-Rich: Watermelon contains antioxidants like vitamin C, vitamin A, and lycopene, which help protect cells from damage, reduce inflammation, and support overall health.

- May Help Lower Blood Pressure: The citrulline in watermelon may help regulate blood pressure and improve cardiovascular health.

- Supports Healthy Digestion: Watermelon contains fiber and water, making it a great choice for supporting healthy digestion and preventing constipation.

- May Help Reduce Muscle Soreness: The citrulline in watermelon may help reduce muscle soreness and improve athletic performance.

- Low in Calories: Watermelon sorbet is a low-calorie dessert option, making it a great choice for those watching their weight.

- Supports Healthy Immune Function: Watermelon contains vitamin C, which is essential for healthy immune function and may help reduce the severity of colds and flu.

- May Help Reduce Inflammation: The antioxidants and anti-inflammatory compounds in watermelon may help reduce inflammation and improve overall health.

Enjoy your watermelon sorbet, a refreshing and nutritious treat.

5. FRUIT KABOBS WITH YOGURT DIP:

 Skewer a variety of fresh fruits such as strawberries, kiwi, pineapple, and grapes on wooden skewers, then serve with a side of Greek yogurt mixed with honey for dipping for a fun and healthy dessert option.
Fruit kabobs with yogurt dip are a fun and healthy dessert option! Here's a simple recipe to make this colorful and delicious treat:

Ingredients:

For the fruit kabobs:
- 1 cup of freshly plucked and cut strawberries
- 1 cup fresh kiwi, peeled and sliced
- 1 cup fresh pineapple, chunks
- 1 cup fresh grapes, halved
- 10-12 wooden skewers

For the yogurt dip:
- 1 cup Greek yogurt
- 2 tablespoons honey
- 1 tablespoon lemon juice (optional)

Instructions:

1. Thread the fresh fruits onto the wooden skewers.

2. In a small bowl, mix together the Greek yogurt, honey, and lemon juice (if using).

3. Serve the fruit kabobs with the yogurt dip on the side.

4. Enjoy!

Tips:

- Use a variety of colorful fruits to make the kabobs visually appealing.

- Adjust the amount of honey to your taste.

- Add a sprinkle of granola or chopped nuts to the yogurt dip for extra crunch.

- Experiment with different types of yogurt, like coconut or almond yogurt, for a unique flavor twist.

Fruit Kabobs with Yogurt Dip is a delicious and nutritious snack that offers several health benefits. Here are some of the benefits:

- Antioxidant-Rich: The various fruits on the kabobs (such as strawberries, grapes, and pineapple) are packed with antioxidants, which help protect cells from damage, reduce inflammation, and support overall health.

- High in Fiber: The fruits and yogurt dip are good sources of dietary fiber, which can help regulate bowel movements, prevent constipation, and support healthy digestion.

- Protein-Rich: The yogurt dip provides protein, which supports muscle growth and repair, and can help regulate appetite and weight.

- May Help Support Healthy Blood Sugar Levels: The fiber and antioxidants in the fruit and yogurt may help regulate blood sugar levels and improve insulin sensitivity.

- Supports Healthy Bones: The yogurt dip is a good source of calcium, vitamin D, and potassium, which are essential for bone health.

- Low in Calories: Fruit kabobs with yogurt dip are a low-calorie snack option, making them a great choice for those watching their weight.

- Supports Healthy Gut Bacteria: The prebiotic fiber in the fruit and yogurt can help feed good gut bacteria, supporting a healthy gut microbiome.

- May Help Reduce Inflammation: The antioxidants and anti-inflammatory compounds in the fruit and yogurt may help reduce inflammation and improve overall health.

Enjoy your fruit kabobs with yogurt dip, a delicious and nutritious snack.

CHAPTER 7

QUICK AND EASY MEALS

1. 30-MINUTE PLANT-BASED MEALS

1. VEGGIE STIR-FRY:

Sauté your favorite vegetables with tofu or tempeh in a flavorful sauce, and serve over cooked rice or noodles for a quick and nutritious meal.

Here's a 30-minute recipe for a delicious veggie stir-fry:

Ingredients:

- 1 cup firm tofu or tempeh, cut into small pieces
- 2 cups mixed vegetables (bell peppers, broccoli, carrots, mushrooms, snow peas)
- 2 tablespoons vegetable oil
- 2 cloves garlic, minced
- 1 tablespoon soy sauce (or stir-fry sauce)

- 1 tablespoon honey

- 1 teaspoon grated ginger

- Salt and pepper, to taste

- Cooked rice or noodles, for serving

Instructions:

1. Prepare ingredients (5 minutes):

    - Cut vegetables into bite-sized pieces.

    - Mince garlic and grate ginger.

2. Cook tofu or tempeh (5 minutes):

    - In a pan, heat up one tablespoon of oil over medium-high heat.

    - Add tofu or tempeh and cook until golden brown on all sides.

    - Take out and place aside from the skillet..

3. Cook vegetables (10 minutes):

    - Pour the last tablespoon of oil into the same pan.   -

- Cook for a minute after adding the garlic and ginger.

    - Add mixed vegetables and cook until tender-crisp.

4. Add sauce and combine (5 minutes):

    - In a small bowl, whisk together soy sauce, honey, and a pinch of salt and pepper.

    - Pour sauce into the pan and stir to coat vegetables.

- Add cooked tofu or tempeh back into the pan and stir to combine.

5. Serve (5 minutes):

    - Serve veggie stir-fry over cooked rice or noodles.

    - Enjoy your quick and nutritious meal!

Timing:

- Prep: 5 minutes

- Cook tofu/tempeh: 5 minutes

- Cook vegetables: 10 minutes

- Add sauce and combine: 5 minutes

- Serve: 5 minutes

- Total: 30 minutes

Enjoy your delicious veggie stir-fry!

Veggie Stir-Fry is a nutritious and delicious meal option that offers numerous health benefits.

Here are some of the benefits:

- High in Vitamins and Minerals: The various vegetables in the stir-fry (such as broccoli, bell peppers, and carrots) are rich in vitamins A, C, and K, and minerals like potassium and iron.

- Antioxidant-Rich: The vegetables in the stir-fry are packed with antioxidants, which help protect cells from damage, reduce inflammation, and support overall health.

- May Help Reduce Chronic Disease Risk: The antioxidants, fiber, and healthy fats in the stir-fry may help reduce the risk of chronic diseases like heart disease, diabetes, and certain cancers.

- Supports Healthy Digestion: The fiber in the vegetables can help regulate bowel movements, prevent constipation, and support healthy digestion.

- May Help Support Healthy Weight: The fiber and water content in the vegetables can help regulate appetite and support healthy weight management.

- Supports Healthy Bones: The vegetables in the stir-fry are rich in calcium, vitamin K, and potassium, which are essential for bone health.

- Low in Calories: Veggie stir-fry is a low-calorie meal option, making it a great choice for those watching their weight.

- Supports Healthy Gut Bacteria: The prebiotic fiber in the vegetables can help feed good gut bacteria, supporting a healthy gut microbiome.

Enjoy your veggie stir-fry, a delicious and nutritious meal.

2. CHICKPEA CURRY:

Simmer chickpeas with canned tomatoes, coconut milk, and curry spices, and serve over quinoa or rice for a satisfying and flavorful dinner.

Here's a 30-minute recipe for a delicious chickpea curry:

Ingredients:
- 1 can chickpeas (14 oz)
- 1 can diced tomatoes (14 oz)

- 1 cup coconut milk

- 2 teaspoons curry powder

- 1 teaspoon ground cumin

- 1/2 teaspoon turmeric

- 1/2 teaspoon cayenne pepper (optional)

- Salt and pepper, to taste

- 2 tablespoons vegetable oil

- Fresh cilantro, for garnish

- Cooked quinoa or rice, for serving

Instructions:

1. Prepare ingredients (5 minutes):

    - Drain and rinse chickpeas.

    - Measure out spices and coconut milk.

2. Sauté onions and spices (5 minutes):

    - In a big pan, warm up the oil over medium heat.

    - Add onions and cook until softened (3-4 minutes).

    - Add curry powder, cumin, turmeric, and cayenne
pepper (if using). Cook for 1 minute.

3. Simmer curry (15 minutes):

    - Combine chickpeas, diced tomatoes, and coconut
milk. Stir to combine.

- Bring to a simmer, then reduce heat and let cook for 15 minutes or until flavors have melded together.

4. Season and serve (5 minutes):

    - Season with salt and pepper to taste.

    - Serve curry over quinoa or rice.

    - Add fresh cilantro as a garnish if you'd like.

Timing:

- Prep: 5 minutes

- Sauté onions and spices: 5 minutes

- Simmer curry: 15 minutes

- Season and serve: 5 minutes

- Total: 30 minutes

Chickpea Curry is a popular and nutritious dish that offers numerous health benefits. It's a great source of protein, fiber, and antioxidants, making it an excellent addition to a healthy diet.

Here are some of the key health benefits of Chickpea Curry:

- Protein Power: Chickpeas are a great source of protein, which helps build and repair muscles, organs, and tissues. Protein also helps regulate appetite, reduce cravings, and support weight management.

- Fiber Rich: Chickpeas are high in dietary fiber, which supports healthy digestion, prevents constipation, and regulates bowel movements. Fiber also helps lower cholesterol levels, manage blood sugar levels, and support healthy weight management.

- Antioxidant Boost: The spices and herbs in the curry, such as turmeric, cumin, and coriander, are packed with antioxidants that protect cells from damage, reduce inflammation, and support overall health. Antioxidants also help reduce the risk of chronic diseases like heart disease, cancer, and cognitive decline.

- Inflammation Reduction: The curcumin in turmeric has potent anti-inflammatory properties that may help reduce inflammation, improve symptoms of arthritis, and support overall health.

- Blood Sugar Management: The fiber and protein in the curry may help regulate blood sugar levels, improve insulin sensitivity, and support healthy weight management.

- Heart Health: The fiber, protein, and antioxidants in the curry may help lower cholesterol levels, regulate blood pressure, and support overall heart health.

- Bone Health: Chickpeas are a good source of calcium, vitamin K, and potassium, which are essential for bone health and may help reduce the risk of osteoporosis.

- Immune System Support: The antioxidants and other compounds in the curry may help boost the immune system, reduce the risk of illnesses, and support overall health.

Enjoy your delicious and nutritious Chickpea Curry.

3. PASTA PRIMAVERA:

Cook your favorite pasta and toss it with sautéed vegetables, garlic, and herbs for a quick and easy plant-based meal.

Here's a 30-minute recipe for Pasta Primavera:

Ingredients:

- 8 oz pasta (linguine or fettuccine work well)
- 2 cups mixed spring vegetables (cherry tomatoes, bell peppers, broccoli, carrots, snap peas)
- 3 cloves garlic, minced
- 1/4 cup olive oil
- 2 tablespoons chopped fresh herbs (basil, parsley, or dill)
- Salt and pepper, to taste
- Grated nutmeg or lemon zest, optional

Instructions:

1. Cook pasta (8-10 minutes):
   - Simmer water with salt until it boils.
  - Cook the pasta until it reaches the desired doneness, as directed on the package.

- Reserve 1 cup pasta water before draining.

2. Sauté vegetables (8-10 minutes):

   - In a big skillet, warm up the olive oil over medium-high heat.

   - Cook for one minute after adding the garlic.

- Add mixed vegetables and cook until tender-crisp.

3. Combine pasta and vegetables (5 minutes):

   - Add cooked pasta to the skillet with vegetables.

   - Mix well, adding more pasta water from the pot if necessary.

   - Season with salt, pepper, and herbs.

4. Serve and enjoy (5 minutes):

   - Serve hot, garnished with additional herbs or a sprinkle of nutmeg or lemon zest if desired.

Timing:

- Cook pasta: 8-10 minutes

- Sauté vegetables: 8-10 minutes

- Combine pasta and vegetables: 5 minutes

- Serve and enjoy: 5 minutes

- Total: 30 minutes

Pasta Primavera is a nutritious and delicious dish that offers numerous health benefits. It's a great source of complex carbohydrates, protein, fiber, and antioxidants.

Here are some of the key health benefits of Pasta Primavera:

- Complex Carbohydrates: Pasta is a good source of complex carbohydrates, which provide sustained energy and support healthy digestion.

- Protein Power: The vegetables and cheese in Pasta Primavera are good sources of protein, which helps build and repair muscles, organs, and tissues.

- Fiber Rich: The vegetables in Pasta Primavera are high in dietary fiber, which supports healthy digestion, prevents constipation, and regulates bowel movements.

- Antioxidant Boost: The vegetables and herbs in Pasta Primavera are packed with antioxidants that protect cells from damage, reduce inflammation, and support overall health.

- Vitamin and Mineral Rich: Pasta Primavera is a good source of vitamins A, C, and K, and minerals like potassium, magnesium, and iron.

- Supports Healthy Weight: The fiber, protein, and complex carbohydrates in Pasta Primavera can help regulate appetite, reduce cravings, and support healthy weight management.

- Supports Healthy Blood Sugar Levels: The fiber and protein in Pasta Primavera may help regulate blood sugar levels and improve insulin sensitivity.

- Supports Healthy Gut Bacteria: The prebiotic fiber in Pasta Primavera can help feed good gut bacteria, supporting a healthy gut microbiome.

Enjoy your delicious and nutritious Pasta Primavera.

4. BLACK BEAN TACOS:

Fill tortillas with seasoned black beans, avocado, salsa, and your favorite toppings for a delicious and filling dinner that's ready in minutes.

Here's a 30-minute recipe for Black Bean Tacos:

Ingredients:

- 1 rinsed and drained can of black beans
- 1 tablespoon olive oil
- 1 small onion, diced
- 1 clove garlic, minced
- 1 packet taco seasoning
- 4 tacos shells
- Avocado, sliced
- Salsa
- Shredded cheese (optional)
- Cilantro, chopped (optional)
- Other desired toppings (diced tomatoes, shredded lettuce, diced bell peppers)

Instructions:

1. Cook black beans (10 minutes):

   - Put oil in a skillet and set it over medium heat.

   - Toss in the garlic and onion and sauté until delicately cooked.

   - Add black beans and taco seasoning. Cook according to package instructions.

2. Prepare toppings (5 minutes):

   - Slice avocado.

   - Prepare salsa and other desired toppings.

3. Assemble tacos (5 minutes):

   - Warm tacos shells according to package instructions.

   - Fill with black beans, avocado, salsa, and desired toppings.

4. Serve and enjoy (5 minutes):

   - Serve immediately and enjoy!

Timing:

- Cook black beans: 10 minutes

- Prepare toppings: 5 minutes

- Assemble tacos: 5 minutes

- Serve and enjoy: 5 minutes

- Total: 30 minutes

Black Bean Tacos are a nutrient-dense food that offers numerous health benefits due to the high content of fiber, protein, antioxidants, and essential vitamins and minerals.
Here are some of the key benefits:

- Fiber Content: Black beans are rich in dietary fiber, containing both soluble and insoluble fiber. The fiber helps regulate bowel movements, prevent constipation, and support healthy gut bacteria.

- Protein Power: Black beans are an excellent source of plant-based protein, essential for building and repairing muscles, organs, and tissues.

- Antioxidant Properties: Black beans contain a range of antioxidants, including polyphenols and flavonoids, which help protect cells from damage, reduce inflammation, and support overall health.

- Heart Health: The fiber, protein, and antioxidants in black beans help lower cholesterol levels, regulate blood pressure, and improve overall cardiovascular health.

- Blood Sugar Control: The fiber and protein in black beans help regulate blood sugar levels and improve insulin sensitivity, making them an excellent choice for those with diabetes or prediabetes.

- Healthy Gut Bacteria: The prebiotic fiber in black beans feeds good gut bacteria, supporting a healthy gut microbiome and boosting the immune system.

- Weight Management: Black beans are low in calories and high in fiber and protein, making them an excellent addition to a weight loss diet.

- Essential Vitamins and Minerals: Black beans are a good source of essential vitamins and minerals like folate, magnesium, and potassium, which support healthy cell growth, blood pressure regulation, and muscle function.

Black Bean Tacos are a nutritious and delicious option that offers numerous health benefits, making them an excellent addition to a balanced diet.

5. QUINOA SALAD:

Mix cooked quinoa with chopped vegetables, beans, herbs, and a simple vinaigrette dressing for a nutritious and satisfying meal that's perfect for lunch or dinner.

Here's a 30-minute recipe for Quinoa Salad:

Ingredients:
- 1 cup quinoa, rinsed and drained
- 2 cups water or vegetable broth
- 1 cup mixed vegetables (cherry tomatoes, cucumber, bell peppers, carrots)
- 1 cup cooked beans (black beans, chickpeas, or kidney beans)
- 1/4 cup chopped fresh herbs (parsley, basil, or cilantro)
- 2 tablespoons simple vinaigrette dressing
- Salt and pepper, to taste
- Optional: avocado, nuts, or seeds for added creaminess and crunch

Instructions:
1. Cook quinoa (15 minutes):

- Heat up some broth or water to a boil.

 - When the quinoa is tender, add it, cover, lower the heat, and simmer.

2. Prepare vegetables and beans (5 minutes):

    - Chop vegetables and beans.

3. Mix quinoa salad (5 minutes):

    - In a large bowl, combine cooked quinoa, vegetables, beans, and herbs.

4. Add dressing and season (5 minutes):

    - Pour vinaigrette dressing over the quinoa mixture and toss to coat.

    - Season with salt and pepper to taste.

5. Serve and enjoy (5 minutes):

    - Serve immediately, garnished with avocado, nuts, or seeds if desired.

Timing:

- Cook quinoa: 15 minutes

- Prepare vegetables and beans: 5 minutes

- Mix quinoa salad: 5 minutes

- Add dressing and season: 5 minutes

- Serve and enjoy: 5 minutes

- Total: 30 minutes

Quinoa Salad is a nutrient-dense food that offers numerous health benefits due to the high content of protein, fiber, antioxidants, and essential vitamins and minerals.

Here are some of the key benefits:

- Protein Power: Quinoa is a complete protein, containing all nine essential amino acids that the body cannot produce on its own.
- Fiber Content: Quinoa is high in dietary fiber, which helps regulate bowel movements, prevent constipation, and support healthy gut bacteria.

- Antioxidant Properties: Quinoa contains various antioxidants like vitamin E and manganese, which help protect cells from damage, reduce inflammation, and support overall health.

- Gluten-Free: Quinoa is gluten-free, making it an excellent option for those with gluten intolerance or celiac disease.

- Heart Health: The fiber, protein, and antioxidants in quinoa help lower cholesterol levels, regulate blood pressure, and improve overall cardiovascular health.

- Blood Sugar Control: Quinoa's fiber and protein help regulate blood sugar levels and improve insulin sensitivity.

- Healthy Gut Bacteria: Quinoa's prebiotic fiber feeds good gut bacteria, supporting a healthy gut microbiome and boosting the immune system.

- Weight Management: Quinoa is low in calories and high in fiber and protein, making it an excellent addition to a weight loss diet.

- Essential Vitamins and Minerals: Quinoa is a good source of essential vitamins and minerals like iron, magnesium, and potassium, which support healthy cell growth, blood pressure regulation, and muscle function.

Quinoa Salad is a nutritious and delicious option that offers numerous health benefits, making it an excellent addition to a balanced diet.

2. ONE-POT WONDERS FOR BUSY NIGHTS

1. LENTIL SOUP:

 Simmer lentils with diced vegetables, vegetable broth, and spices in a large pot until tender for a hearty and comforting meal that's ready in no time.

Servings: 4-6 people

Cooking Time: 30 minutes

Ingredients:

- 1 cup dried green or brown lentils, rinsed and drained
- 4 cups vegetable broth
- 1 large onion, diced
- 2 cloves garlic, minced
- 2 carrots, peeled and diced
- 1 celery stalk, diced
- 1 can diced tomatoes (14.5 oz)
- 1 teaspoon dried thyme
- 1 teaspoon dried rosemary
- 1 bay leaf

- Salt and pepper, to taste

- Optional: lemon juice, red pepper flakes, kale or spinach

Instructions:

Step 1: Saute the Aromatics (5 minutes)

1. In a large pot set over medium heat, warm up two tablespoons of olive oil.
2. Add the diced onion, minced garlic, carrots, and celery.
3. Cook until the vegetables are tender, about 5 minutes.

Step 2: Add Lentils and Broth (10 minutes)

1. Add the rinsed lentils, vegetable broth, diced tomatoes, thyme, rosemary, and bay leaf.
2. Season with salt and pepper to taste.
3. After bringing the mixture to a boil, lower the heat and let it simmer.

Step 3: Simmer the Soup (15 minutes)

1. Let the soup simmer for 15 minutes, or until the lentils are tender.
2. Check for seasoning and adjust as needed.

Step 4: Serve and Enjoy!

1. Serve hot, garnished with chopped fresh herbs or a squeeze of lemon juice (optional).
2. Enjoy with crusty bread or a side salad.

Tips and Variations:

- Squeeze in some lemon juice for a zesty taste explosion.
- Spice it up with red pepper flakes or a diced jalapeno.
- Mix in some chopped kale or spinach for an extra nutritional boost.
- Serve with a swirl of olive oil and a side of crusty bread.

Lentil Soup is a nutritious and delicious option that offers numerous health benefits due to the high content of protein, fiber, antioxidants, and essential vitamins and minerals in lentils.

Here are some of the key benefits:

- High in Protein: Lentils are a great source of plant-based protein, essential for building and repairing muscles, organs, and tissues.

- Rich in Fiber: Lentils are high in dietary fiber, which helps regulate bowel movements, prevent constipation, and support healthy gut bacteria.

- Antioxidant Properties: Lentils contain antioxidants like polyphenols and flavonoids, which help protect cells from damage, reduce inflammation, and support overall health.

- Low in Calories: Lentils are relatively low in calories, making them an excellent addition to a weight loss diet.

- Supports Heart Health: The fiber, protein, and antioxidants in lentils help lower cholesterol levels, regulate blood pressure, and improve overall cardiovascular health.

- Helps Regulate Blood Sugar: Lentils' fiber and protein help regulate blood sugar levels and improve insulin sensitivity.

- Supports Healthy Gut Bacteria: Lentils' prebiotic fiber feeds good gut bacteria, supporting a healthy gut microbiome and boosting the immune system.

- Rich in Essential Vitamins and Minerals: Lentils are a good source of essential vitamins and minerals like iron, potassium, and phosphorus, which support healthy cell growth, blood pressure regulation, and muscle function.

Lentil Soup is a nutritious and delicious option that offers numerous health benefits, making it an excellent addition to a balanced diet.

2. ONE-POT PASTA:

Cook pasta with canned tomatoes, vegetables, and herbs in one pot for a flavorful and fuss-free dinner that requires minimal cleanup.
Here's a step-by-step guide to cooking a delicious plant-based one-pot pasta:

Cooking Time: 25-30 minutes

 Ingredients:

- 8 oz pasta of your choice (e.g., penne, rotini, or rigatoni)
- 2 cups canned crushed tomatoes
- 1 cup mixed vegetables (e.g., cherry tomatoes, sliced bell peppers, diced zucchini)
- 2 cloves garlic, minced
- 1 cup vegetable broth
- 1 tablespoon olive oil
- 1 teaspoon dried basil
- 1 teaspoon dried oregano
- Salt and pepper, to taste
- Fresh parsley or basil, chopped (optional)

Instructions:

Step 1: Prepare the Pot

1. Choose a large pot (at least 3-4 quarts) with a heavy bottom (e.g., stainless steel or ceramic).
2. Add the olive oil and swirl it around to coat the bottom.

Step 2: Sauté the Garlic and Vegetables

1. Add the minced garlic and sauté for 1-2 minutes until fragrant.
2. Add the mixed vegetables and cook for 3-4 minutes until they start to soften.

Step 3: Add the Tomato Mixture

1. Pour in the canned crushed tomatoes, vegetable broth, dried basil, and dried oregano.
2. Stir well to combine.

Step 4: Add the Pasta

1. Add the pasta to the pot, making sure it's fully submerged in the tomato mixture.
2. Stir gently to prevent the pasta from sticking together.

Step 5: Simmer and Cook

1. Bring the mixture to a simmer.
2. Reduce the heat to medium-low and let cook for 15-20 minutes or until the pasta is al dente.
3. Adjust the seasoning with salt and pepper to taste.

Step 6: Serve and Enjoy!

1. Serve hot, garnished with chopped fresh parsley or basil if desired.
2. Enjoy your delicious plant-based one-pot pasta!

This recipe is not only flavorful but also easy to prepare and requires minimal cleanup. The best part? You can customize it with your favorite vegetables and herbs to make it your own!

One-Pot Pasta is a nutrient-dense meal that offers numerous health benefits due to its combination of whole grains, protein, vegetables, and healthy fats.

Here are some of the main advantages:

- Whole Grain Goodness: Whole grain pasta provides sustained energy, fiber, and essential vitamins and minerals like iron, B vitamins, and selenium.

- Protein Powerhouse: The pasta sauce's protein content from lean ground meat, beans, or lentils helps build and repair muscles, organs, and tissues.

- Vegetable Bonanza: The variety of colorful vegetables in the sauce, such as tomatoes, bell peppers, and onions, provides a range of antioxidants, vitamins, and minerals.

- Healthy Fat Benefits: Olive oil and other healthy fats in the sauce support heart health, reduce inflammation, and aid in the absorption of vitamins and minerals.

- Fiber Frenzy: The combination of whole grains and vegetables provides a good amount of fiber, supporting healthy digestion, bowel movements, and satiety.

- Antioxidant Boost: The various vegetables and tomatoes in the sauce contain antioxidants that help protect cells from damage, reduce inflammation, and support overall health.

- Supports Healthy Weight: One-Pot Pasta's balanced mix of protein, fiber, and healthy fats helps regulate appetite, reduce cravings, and support weight management.

- Convenient and Nutritious: One-Pot Pasta is a quick and easy meal option that still provides a wealth of nutritional benefits, making it an excellent addition to a balanced diet.

One-Pot Pasta is a nutritious and delicious meal that offers numerous health benefits, making it an excellent choice for those looking for a convenient and healthy meal option.

3. VEGETABLE CURRY:

Combine diced vegetables, canned chickpeas, coconut milk, and curry paste in a pot, and simmer until vegetables are tender for a flavorful and aromatic curry dish.
Here are the instructions to cook a delicious Vegetable Curry:

Heat 2 tablespoons of oil in a large pot over medium heat.

Add 1 onion, diced, and cook until softened, about 5 minutes.

Add 2 cloves of garlic, minced, and 1-inch piece of ginger, grated, and cook for another minute.

Stir in 2 tablespoons of curry paste and cook for 1-2 minutes, until fragrant.

Add 2 cups of mixed vegetables (such as bell peppers, carrots, potatoes, and zucchini) and cook for 5 minutes, stirring occasionally.

Add 1 can of chickpeas (14 oz), 1 cup of coconut milk, and 1 cup of vegetable broth. Stir well to combine.

Bring the mixture to a simmer, then reduce the heat to low and cook, covered, until the vegetables are tender, about 20-25 minutes.

Season with salt and pepper to taste.

Serve hot over rice or with naan bread, garnished with fresh herbs, if desired.

Enjoy your flavorful and aromatic Vegetable Curry! Vegetable Curry is a nutritious and delicious option that offers numerous health benefits due to the variety of vegetables and spices used in its preparation.

Here are some of the main advantages:

- Antioxidant Rich: The various vegetables used in the curry, such as bell peppers, carrots, and potatoes, provide a range of antioxidants that help protect cells from damage and reduce inflammation.

- Anti-Inflammatory Effects: The spices used in the curry, such as turmeric, cumin, and coriander, have anti-inflammatory properties that may help reduce the risk of chronic diseases like heart disease and cancer.

- Fiber Content: The vegetables and legumes used in the curry provide a good amount of fiber, supporting healthy digestion, bowel movements, and satiety.

- Vitamin and Mineral Rich: The vegetables and spices in the curry provide a range of essential vitamins and minerals like vitamin A, vitamin C, calcium, and iron.

- Supports Healthy Gut Bacteria: The prebiotic fiber in the vegetables and legumes helps feed good gut bacteria, supporting a healthy gut microbiome.

- May Help Reduce Chronic Disease Risk: The antioxidants, anti-inflammatory compounds, and fiber in the curry may help reduce the risk of chronic diseases like heart disease, diabetes, and certain cancers.

- Supports Healthy Weight: The balanced mix of protein, fiber, and healthy fats in the curry helps regulate appetite, reduce cravings, and support weight management.

- Convenient and Nutritious: Vegetable Curry is a quick and easy meal option that still provides a wealth of nutritional benefits, making it an excellent addition to a balanced diet.

Vegetable Curry is a nutritious and delicious meal that offers numerous health benefits, making it an excellent choice for those looking for a convenient and healthy meal option.

3. MEAL PREP TIPS FOR EFFORTLESS EATING

1. PLAN AHEAD:

Take some time each week to plan your meals and create a shopping list to ensure you have everything you need for quick and easy meals.

Planning ahead is a crucial step in meal prep that saves time and stress in the long run. The following advice will help you make an efficient plan:

- Set a specific day and time each week to plan your meals, e.g., Sunday evening.
- Consider your schedule for the upcoming week and plan meals that fit your busy days.
- Choose recipes that can be cooked in bulk and reheated throughout the week.
- Make a list of the ingredients you need and check what you already have in your pantry, fridge, and freezer.
- Make a shopping list and follow it to prevent impulsive purchases.
- Consider meal prepping with a friend or family member to split ingredients and cooking duties.

- Keep your meal plans flexible in case your schedule changes or you need to swap out ingredients.
- Use a meal planning app or website to help you organize your plans and grocery lists.

By planning, you'll be able to:

- Save time when you're busy during the workweek.
- Avoid last-minute takeout or fast food
- Stay on track with your dietary goals
- Reduce food waste
- Enjoy stress-free meal times

Remember, meal prep is all about finding a system that works for you and making healthy eating easier and more enjoyable!

Cook large batches of grains, beans, and vegetables ahead of time and store them in the fridge or freezer for easy meal prep throughout the week.

During meal prep, batch cooking is a fantastic method to save time and effort! By cooking large batches of staple ingredients like grains, beans, and vegetables, you can create a treasure trove of ready-to-use ingredients for quick and easy meals throughout the week.

The following advice can help with batch cooking:

- Choose ingredients that freeze well, like rice, quinoa, lentils, chickpeas, and roasted vegetables.
- Cook large batches on the weekend or a day off, when you have more time.
- Portion the cooked ingredients into individual servings or family-sized portions and store them in:
    - Refrigerate airtight containers for a maximum of five days; use freezer-safe bags or containers for a maximum of three months.
- Label and date each container or bag so you can easily keep track of what you have and how long it's been stored.

- Use your batch-cooked ingredients to whip up quick meals like salads, bowls, stir-fries, and soups.
- Get creative and experiment with different seasonings and spices to add flavor to your batch-cooked ingredients.

Some popular batch cooking ideas include:

- Cooking a big pot of rice or quinoa and using it throughout the week in different meals
- Roasting a large tray of vegetables like broccoli, sweet potatoes, or cauliflower and using them in salads, bowls, or as a side dish
- Cooking a large batch of lentils or chickpeas and using them in soups, salads, or as a protein source in meals

By batch cooking, you'll save time during the week, reduce food waste, and have healthy ingredients on hand to fuel your body!

3. PREP INGREDIENTS:

Wash, chop, and portion out fruits and vegetables ahead of time so they're ready to go when you need them for cooking or snacking.

Prepping ingredients is a great way to make healthy eating easier and more convenient! By washing, chopping, and portioning out fruits and vegetables ahead of time, you can:

- Save time when preparing and cooking meals.
- Encourage healthy snacking
- Reduce food waste by using up fresh ingredients before they go bad
- Make meal planning and grocery shopping easier by having a stash of prepped ingredients to draw from

Here are some tips for prepping ingredients:

- Set aside time each week (e.g., Sunday evening) to prep ingredients for the next few days
- Choose fruits and vegetables that keep well when chopped and stored (e.g., berries, citrus fruits, carrots, bell peppers)

- Wash and dry ingredients thoroughly before chopping and storing
- Use airtight containers or bags to store prepped ingredients in the fridge
- Label and date containers so you know what you have and how long it's been stored
- Consider prepping ingredients like:
    - Leafy greens (wash, dry, and chop for salads or sautés)
    - Herbs (chop and store in airtight containers for fresh flavor)
    - Vegetables (chop and store in airtight containers for snacking or cooking)
    - Fruits (wash, chop, and store in airtight containers for snacking or adding to oatmeal or yogurt)

By prepping ingredients ahead of time, you'll make healthy eating easier, save time, and reduce stress in the kitchen!

Stock your pantry with canned beans, diced tomatoes, frozen vegetables, and pre-cooked grains for quick and convenient meal prep.

Using convenience foods can be a great way to save time and effort in meal prep! Stocking your pantry with items like:

- Canned beans (black beans, chickpeas, kidney beans)
- Diced tomatoes
- Frozen vegetables (broccoli, cauliflower, berries)
- Pre-cooked grains (quinoa, brown rice, lentils)

can help you whip up quick and healthy meals. These foods are often:

- Already prepped (washed, chopped, cooked)
- Shelf-stable or frozen for long-term storage
- Easy to incorporate into a variety of dishes

Using convenience foods can:
- Spend less time preparing and cooking meals.
- Make healthy eating simpler and more accessible

- Cut down on food waste by using up ingredients before they go bad
- Be an economical way to stock your pantry

Some tips for using convenience foods:

- Choose options that are low in added salt, sugar, and unhealthy fats
- Check expiration dates and store properly to maintain freshness
- Use them as a starting point and add your fresh ingredients to enhance flavor and nutrition
- Get creative and experiment with different combinations to keep meals interesting!

By incorporating convenience foods into your meal prep routine, you can make healthy eating easier, faster, and more enjoyable!

5. PACK PORTABLE SNACKS:

Prepare snacks like trail mix, energy balls, and chopped fruits and vegetables to take with you on the go for easy and healthy eating throughout the day.

Packing portable snacks is a great way to ensure healthy eating even when you're away from home! Preparing snacks like:
- Trail mix with nuts, seeds, and dried fruits
- Energy balls consisting of honey, nut butter, and oats
- Chopped fruits and vegetables like carrots, apples, and berries can provide a quick and easy energy boost whenever you need it. These snacks are:

- Easy to prepare in advance
- Lightweight and easy to pack in a bag or container
- Nutrient-dense to keep you satisfied and focused
- can be altered to accommodate your dietary requirements and tastes

Packing portable snacks can:

- Help you avoid relying on fast food or vending machine snacks

- Save you money by reducing the need for last-minute takeout or coffee shop treats
- Support your overall health and well-being

Some tips for packing portable snacks:
- Choose snacks that are non-perishable or can be stored at room temperature
- Pack them in reusable containers or bags to reduce waste
- Consider portioning out individual servings to avoid overeating
- Get creative and experiment with new ingredients and recipes to keep your snacks interesting!

CHAPTER 8

SPECIAL OCCASION FEASTS

1. ELEGANT ENTERTAINING WITH PLANT-BASED CUISINE

1. STUFFED PORTOBELLO MUSHROOMS:

Fill large portobello mushroom caps with a savory mixture of quinoa, vegetables, and herbs, then bake until tender and golden for an impressive and delicious appetizer or main course.

Here are the instructions to cook Stuffed Portobello Mushrooms:

Ingredients:

- 4 large portobello mushroom caps
- 1 cup quinoa, rinsed and drained
- 2 cups water or vegetable broth
- 1 tablespoon olive oil

- 1 onion, finely chopped

- 2 cloves garlic, minced

- 1 cup mixed vegetables (such as bell peppers, carrots, and zucchini)

- 2 teaspoons dried thyme

- 1 teaspoon dried rosemary

- Salt and pepper, to taste

- 1/4 cup nutritional yeast (optional)

Instructions:

1. Preheat the oven to 375°F (190°C).

2. In a medium saucepan, bring the quinoa and water or broth to a boil. Reduce the heat to low, cover, and cook for 15-20 minutes, or as long as the quinoa is tender and the liquid has been absorbed.

3. While the quinoa is cooking, heat the olive oil in a large skillet over medium heat. Cook the onion and garlic, mixing occasionally, till the onion is translucent, about five minutes.

4. Add the mixed vegetables, thyme, and rosemary to the skillet. Cook while mixing occasionally, until the veggies are tender, around five to seven minutes.

5. Stir in the cooked quinoa, salt, and pepper.

6. Wipe the mushroom caps clean with a damp cloth and remove the stems.

7. Fill each mushroom cap with the quinoa-vegetable mixture, dividing it evenly among the four mushrooms.

8. If using nutritional yeast, sprinkle it on top of the filling.

9. Place the stuffed mushrooms on a baking sheet lined with parchment paper.

10. Bake for 20-25 minutes, or until the mushrooms are tender and the filling is heated through.

11. Serve hot and enjoy!

Note: Nutritional yeast has a nutty, cheesy flavor and can be used to give the dish a cheesy flavor without the dairy. It's optional, but recommended for an extra burst of flavor.

Stuffed Portobello mushrooms are a mouthwatering treat that combines the meaty flavor of mushrooms with various savory fillings. This delectable duo offers several health benefits:

- Meaty Goodness: Portobello mushrooms have an intense meaty flavor, making them an excellent vegetarian option.

- Umami Flavor: They are rich in umami taste, which is associated with savory and rich flavors.

- Low in Calories: Portobello mushrooms are relatively low in calories, making them a guilt-free treat.

- Versatile: They can be stuffed with various fillings like spinach artichoke, sausage marinara, and cheese, offering diverse flavor profiles.

- Rich in Fiber: Portobello mushrooms contain dietary fiber, supporting healthy digestion and satiety.

- Antioxidant Properties: They contain antioxidants that protect the body from oxidative stress and inflammation.

Some popular fillings for stuffed Portobello mushrooms include:

- Spinach and Artichoke

- Sausage Marinara

- Cheese and Herbs

- Garlic and Lemon

- Mushroom Duxelle

This savory treat is perfect for a quick dinner or as a starter for a dinner party, offering a flavorful and healthy option for various occasions.

2. BUTTERNUT SQUASH RISOTTO:

Cook creamy risotto with roasted butternut squash, vegetable broth, white wine, and aromatics until rich and flavorful for a luxurious and comforting dish that's perfect for special occasions.

Here's a recipe for Butternut Squash Risotto:

Ingredients:
- 8 cups low-sodium chicken or vegetable broth, heated
- 3 tablespoons unsalted butter
- 1 medium butternut squash (roughly 2 1/2 pounds), skinned and cut into half-inch pieces (about 4 cups)
- 1 1/2 tablespoons chopped fresh sage leaves
- 1 teaspoon kosher salt, divided
- 1/2 teaspoon freshly ground black pepper, divided
- 1 large shallot, finely chopped
- 2 cups Arborio rice
- 1/2 cup dry white wine
- 1 cup beautifully grated Parmesan cheese (around two ounces), plus more to serve.

Instructions:

1. Roast the butternut squash with butter, sage, salt and pepper for 10-12 minutes.

2. Sauté shallots and add rice, cooking until edges have turned translucent.

3. Add wine and cook until the liquid has been absorbed.

4. Add the broth one ladle at a time, stirring until almost completely absorbed.

5. Stir in the roasted squash and Parmesan cheese.

6. Season with salt as needed and serve hot.

Butternut squash risotto is a popular Italian-inspired dish that combines the sweetness of butternut squash with the creaminess of risotto. This comforting meal offers several health benefits and flavor variations:

- Rich in Vitamins: Butternut squash is a good source of vitamins A, C, and E, as well as minerals like potassium and magnesium.

- Antioxidant Properties: Butternut squash contains antioxidants that protect the body from oxidative stress and inflammation.

- Comfort Food: Risotto is a comforting and filling base for the dish.

- Versatile: This dish can be made with various fillings like mozzarella, pine nuts, and fresh herbs like sage and rosemary, offering diverse flavor profiles.

- Creamy and Savory: The combination of butternut squash and risotto creates a creamy and savory flavor profile.

Some popular variations of butternut squash risotto include:

- Using different types of cheese like parmesan or mozzarella
- Adding fresh herbs like parsley or sage
- Using various types of squash like acorn or kabocha
- Adding some spice with red pepper flakes

This comforting and flavorful dish is perfect for a cozy night in or a dinner party with friends, offering a delicious and healthy option for various occasions.

3. RATATOUILLE TIAN:

Layer thinly sliced zucchini, yellow squash, eggplant, tomatoes, and onions in a baking dish, then bake until tender and golden for a stunning and flavorful vegetable tian that's sure to impress.

Here's a recipe for Ratatouille Tian:

Ingredients:
- One huge eggplant, cut into quarter-inch thick rounds.
- 2 medium zucchinis, sliced into 1/4-inch thick rounds
- 1 medium yellow squash, sliced into 1/4-inch thick rounds
- 1 big onion, cut into a quarter-inch thick rings
- 3 large tomatoes, sliced into 1/4-inch thick rounds
- 2 cloves garlic, minced
- 2 tablespoons olive oil
- Salt and pepper, to taste
- Fresh basil leaves, chopped (optional)

Instructions:

1. Preheat the oven to 375°F (190°C).
2. In a large bowl, toss together the eggplant zucchini, yellow squash, onion, and tomatoes.

3. In a small bowl, mix the garlic and olive oil.

4. Grease a 9x13-inch baking dish with the garlic oil mixture.

5. Layer the vegetables in the prepared baking dish, overlapping slightly.

6. Sprinkle enough salt and pepper according to your preference.

7. Cover with aluminium foil and bake for thirty minutes.

8. Remove the foil and continue baking for an additional 20-25 minutes, or until the vegetables are tender and golden brown.

9. Sprinkle with chopped basil leaves, if desired.

10. Serve hot and enjoy!

This Ratatouille Tian is a beautiful and delicious way to showcase the flavors of summer vegetables. The layering of the vegetables creates a stunning presentation, and the garlic oil adds a rich and savory flavor. Great for an unforgettable supper at home or a special occasion!

Ratatouille Tian is a classic Provençal dish from France, made with a rich and flavorful vegetable stew topped with a crispy, golden-brown crust. This hearty and aromatic dish offers several health benefits and flavor variations:

- Vegetable-Packed: Ratatouille is a rich source of vitamins, minerals, and antioxidants from the variety of vegetables used, including eggplant, zucchini, bell peppers, and tomatoes.

- Fiber-Rich: The vegetables and whole wheat crust provide a good amount of dietary fiber, supporting healthy digestion and satiety.

- Anti-Inflammatory Properties: The vegetables and herbs used in ratatouille have anti-inflammatory properties, which may help reduce inflammation and improve overall health.

- Versatile: This dish can be made with various vegetables, herbs, and spices, offering diverse flavor profiles.

- Crispy Crust: The Tian's crispy crust adds a satisfying texture and flavor contrast to the soft vegetables.

Some popular variations of Ratatouille Tian include:

- Using different vegetables like mushrooms or fennel
- Including fresh spices, such as parsley or rosemary
- Using various cheeses like goat cheese or parmesan
- Adding some spice with red pepper flakes

This flavorful and nutritious dish is perfect for a cozy dinner or a special occasion, offering a delicious and healthy option for various gatherings.

4. MUSHROOM WELLINGTON:

Wrap savory mushroom duxelles in puff pastry and bake until golden and flaky for an elegant and satisfying main course that's perfect for holiday dinners and celebrations.

Here's a recipe for making Mushroom Wellington:

Ingredients:

- Puff pastry
- Mushrooms
- Onion
- Garlic
- Rosemary
- Pecans
- Olive oil
- Salt
- Pepper
- Sherry vinegar
- Balsamic vinegar
- Egg wash

Instructions:

227

1. Preheat oven to 400 F.

2. Make the filling by sautéing the mushrooms, onions, garlic, salt, and rosemary in olive oil.

3. Add the sherry vinegar, balsamic vinegar, pecans, and pepper to the filling.

4. Let the filling cool.

5. Roll out the puff pastry and place the filling in the center.

6. Roll the pastry up and over the filling and score the pastry.

7. Brush the pastry with egg wash.

8. Bake for 35-40 minutes, or until the pastry is golden brown.

The result is a golden flaky crust filled with earthy savory mushrooms and toasty nutty pecans

Mushroom Wellington is a savory and rich vegetarian main dish that offers several health benefits and flavor variations :

- Rich in Vitamins: Mushrooms are a good source of vitamins A, C, and E, as well as minerals like potassium and magnesium.

228

- Antioxidant Properties: Mushrooms contain antioxidants that protect the body from oxidative stress and inflammation.
- Comfort Food: Wellington is a comforting and filling base for the dish.
- Versatile: This dish can be made with various fillings like leek, garlic, spinach, and thyme.
- Decadent Flavors: The combination of mushroom and leek filling, wrapped in puff pastry, creates a creamy and savory flavor profile.

Some popular variations of Mushroom Wellington include:

- Using different types of mushrooms like portobello or cremini
- Adding some spice with red pepper flakes
- Using various cheeses like goat cheese or blue cheese
- Adding some crunch with nuts like walnuts or cashews
- Making it vegan by using vegan puff pastry and dairy-free cheese

5. CHOCOLATE RASPBERRY TART:

Make a decadent chocolate tart crust filled with creamy chocolate ganache and topped with fresh raspberries for a show-stopping dessert that will delight your guests.

Here's a recipe for making a chocolate raspberry tart [1]:
Ingredients:

Tart Dough:

- Dark Chocolate (with a minimum of 70% cocoa solids)
- Unsalted French Butter
- Heavy Whipping Cream
- Fresh Raspberries
- Powdered Sugar
- Raspberry Glaze

Method:

- Mix the tart ingredients and wrath p in plastic and chill until firm.
- Roll out the dough and press it into the bottom of a tart pan.

- Poke the bottom with a fork and then transfer it to the freezer to chill and rest before baking.
- Pour warmed cream and corn syrup, heated in a small saucepan over medium heat, over melted chocolate, te, and add the butter and raspberry liqueur.
- Pour the chocolate ganache into the cooled tart sheld smooth out the top and allow the chocolate to set.
- Garnish with raspberries and press them into the nearly set chocolate.

Tips:

- Consider the shape of the tart and the arrangement of the raspberries.
- Choose quality ingredients, such as high-quality dark chocolate with a cocoa content of at least 70% and European-style butter.
- Perfect the pastry crust by keeping all ingredients cold before mixing and, handling the dough minimally to prevent overworking it, which can lead to toughness.
- Make a smooth chocolate ganache by heating the cream until it's just hot enough to melt the chocolate and

allowing the chocolate and cream to sit for a few minutes before stirring.

Chocolate Raspberry Tart is a match made in heaven, combining the richness of dark chocolate with the sweet-tartness of fresh raspberries. This decadent dessert is not only a treat for the taste buds but also offers several health benefits.

Raspberries are packed with:
- Vitamin C and manganese for immune function and antioxidant properties
- Fiber for healthy digestion and satiety
- Antioxidants like ellagic acid for anti-inflammatory effects

Dark chocolate contains:
- Flavonoids for heart health and antioxidant properties
- Magnesium for bone health and energy production
- Copper for immune function and connective tissue health

Treat yourself to a slice (or two!) of Chocolate Raspberry Tart and indulge in the sweet and tangy

delight while reaping the benefits of these nutritious
ingredients.

2. HOLIDAY AND CELEBRATION MENUS:

1. THANKSGIVING FEAST:

Start with roasted vegetable soup or salad, followed by stuffed acorn squash or lentil loaf as the main course, and finish with pumpkin pie or apple crisp for a classic and satisfying Thanksgiving meal.

Here are the instructions for cooking a plant-based Thanksgiving feast:

Roasted Vegetable Soup

Ingredients:
- 2 tablespoons olive oil
- 1 onion, chopped
- 3 cloves garlic, minced
- 3 carrots, chopped
- 3 celery stalks, chopped
- 2 potatoes, chopped
- 2 cups vegetable broth
- 1 can diced tomatoes
- 1 teaspoon dried thyme

- Salt and pepper, to taste

Instructions:

1. Preheat the oven to 425°F (220°C).

2. Heat the olive oil in a big pot over a low flame.

3. Add the onion, garlic, carrots, celery, and potatoes. Cook for approximately ten minutes, or till the vegetables are tender.

4. Add the vegetable broth, diced tomatoes, and thyme. Bring to a boil, then transfer to the preheated oven.

5. Roast for 25-30 minutes or until the vegetables are tender.

6. Blend the soup until smooth. Season with salt and pepper to taste.

Stuffed Acorn Squash

Ingredients:

- 2 acorn squash, and cut in half, and seeds taken out
- 1 cup cooked rice
- 1 cup black beans, cooked
- 1 cup diced tomatoes
- 1/4 cup chopped fresh cilantro
- 2 tablespoons olive oil

- 1 teaspoon cumin

- Salt and pepper, to taste

Instructions:

1. Preheat the oven to 400°F (200°C).

2. In a large bowl, combine the cooked rice, black beans, diced tomatoes, cilantro, olive oil, cumin, salt, and pepper.

3. Divide the filling among the squash halves, filling them as full as possible.

4. Place the squash on a baking sheet and bake for 30-40 minutes or until the squash is tender.

Lentil Loaf

Ingredients:
- 1 cup cooked lentils
- 1 cup breadcrumbs
- 1/2 cup chopped onion
- 1/4 cup chopped fresh parsley
- 2 cloves garlic, minced
- 1 tablespoon tomato paste
- 1 teaspoon dried thyme

- 1/4 cup ketchup

- 1/4 cup water

- 1 tablespoon olive oil

- Salt and pepper, to taste

Instructions:

1. Preheat the oven to 375°F (190°C).

2. In a large bowl, combine the cooked lentils, breadcrumbs, onion, parsley, garlic, tomato paste, thyme, ketchup, water, and olive oil.

3. Mix well and transfer the mixture to a loaf pan.

4. Bake for 40-45 minutes or until the loaf is firm and golden brown.

Pumpkin Pie

Ingredients:

- 1 cup pumpkin puree

- 1 cup non-dairy milk

- 1/2 cup sugar

- 1/2 teaspoon salt

- 1/2 teaspoon cinnamon

- 1/4 teaspoon nutmeg

- 1/4 teaspoon ginger

- 2 tablespoons cornstarch

- 1/4 cup non-dairy whipped cream

Instructions:

1. Preheat the oven to 425°F (220°C).

2. In a large bowl, combine the pumpkin puree, non-dairy milk, sugar, salt, cinnamon, nutmeg, and ginger.

3. Mix well and pour into a pie crust.

4. Bake for 15 minutes, then reduce the heat to 350°F (180°C) and bake for an additional 30-40 minutes or until the filling is set.

5. Top with non-dairy whipped cream and serve.

Apple Crisp

Ingredients:

- 6 apples, sliced

- 1/2 cup sugar

- 2 tablespoons flour

- 1 teaspoon cinnamon

- 1/4 teaspoon nutmeg

- 1/4 teaspoon salt

- 1/2 cup non-dairy butter

- 1 cup oatmeal

- 1/2 cup brown sugar

Instructions:

1. Preheat the oven to 375°F (190°C).

2. Put the apple slices, sugar, flour, nutmeg, cinnamon, and salt in a big bowl.

3. Thoroughly stir and move to an oven proof dish.

4. In a separate bowl, combine the non-dairy butter, oatmeal, and brown sugar.

5. Mix well and sprinkle over the apple mixture.

6. Bake for 30-40 minutes or until the apples are tender and the topping is crispy.

Begin with a festive appetizer like stuffed mushrooms or vegan cheese board, then serve roasted vegetable Wellington or stuffed peppers as the main course, and end with a decadent yule log or gingerbread cake for a memorable holiday dinner.

Here are the instructions for cooking a plant-based Christmas dinner:

Stuffed Mushrooms

Ingredients:

- 12 mushrooms, cleaned and stems removed
- 1/2 cup breadcrumbs
- 1/4 cup vegan cheese, crumbled
- 1/4 cup chopped fresh parsley
- 2 cloves garlic, minced
- 1 tablespoon olive oil
- Salt and pepper, to taste

Instructions:

1. Preheat the oven to 375°F (190°C).

2. In a bowl, mix breadcrumbs, vegan cheese, parsley, garlic, and olive oil.

3. Stuff each mushroom with the mixture and bake for 15-20 minutes or until tender.

Vegan Cheese Board

Ingredients:

- Assorted vegan cheeses (e.g., vegan brie, vegan cheddar)
- Crackers or bread
- Fresh fruit (e.g., grapes, berries)
- Nuts (e.g., almonds, walnuts)

Instructions:

1. Arrange the vegan cheeses, crackers, fruit, and nuts on a platter.

2. Serve and enjoy!

Roasted Vegetable Wellington

Ingredients:

- 1 sheet puff pastry, thawed

- One cup of roasted veggies, such as onions, bell peppers, and zucchini
- 1/4 cup vegan cheese, crumbled
- 1 tablespoon olive oil
- Salt and pepper, to taste

Instructions:
1. Preheat the oven to 400°F (200°C).
2. Roll out the puff pastry and place the roasted vegetables and vegan cheese in the center.
3. Brush the edges with olive oil and fold the pastry over the filling.
4. Bake for 25-30 minutes or until golden brown.

Stuffed Peppers

Ingredients:
- 4 bell peppers, any color
- 1 cup cooked rice
- 1 cup black beans, cooked
- 1 cup diced tomatoes
- 1/4 cup chopped fresh cilantro
- 2 tablespoons olive oil

- Salt and pepper, to taste

Instructions:

1. Preheat the oven to 375°F (190°C).

2. Slice off the peppers' tops, then take out the seeds and membranes.

3. Fill each pepper with the rice, black beans, diced tomatoes, and cilantro.

4. Drizzle with olive oil and bake for 25-30 minutes or until tender.

Yule Log

Ingredients:

- 1 cup vegan chocolate cake mix
- 1 cup non-dairy milk
- 1/4 cup vegan butter, melted
- 1 teaspoon vanilla extract
- Powdered sugar, for dusting

Instructions:

1. Preheat the oven to 350°F (180°C).

2. Mir the cake mix, non-dairy milk, melted vegan butter, and vanilla extract.

3. Pour into a log-shaped pan and bake for 25-30 minutes or until a toothpick comes out clean.

4. Dust with powdered sugar and serve.

Gingerbread Cake

Ingredients:

- 1 cup vegan gingerbread cake mix

- 1 cup non-dairy milk

- 1/4 cup vegan butter, melted

- 1 teaspoon vanilla extract

- Powdered sugar, for dusting

Instructions:

1. Preheat the oven to 350°F (180°C).

2. Mir the cake mix, non-dairy milk, melted vegan butter, and vanilla extract.

3. Pour into a greased cake pan and bake for 25-30 minutes or until a toothpick comes out clean.

4. Dust with powdered sugar and serve.

3. NEW YEAR'S EVE PARTY:

Create a spread of elegant appetizers like mini quiches, avocado bruschetta, and stuffed dates, followed by a buffet of pasta dishes, risottos, and stir-fries, and finish with champagne and dessert platters filled with cookies, chocolates, and fruit for a festive and celebratory evening.

Here are the instructions for cooking a plant-based New Year's Eve party meal:

Appetizers:

Mini Quiches:

  - Ingredients: tofu, vegan cheese, bell peppers, onions, mushrooms, spinach
  - Instructions: Preheat oven to 375°F (190°C). Mix tofu, vegan cheese, bell peppers, onions, mushrooms, and spinach. Fill a small muffin tin, then bake for fifteen to twenty minutes.

  Avocado Bruschetta:
  - Ingredients: avocado, cherry tomatoes, basil, garlic, bread

- Instructions: Toast bread and top with mashed avocado, cherry tomatoes, basil, and garlic.

Stuffed Dates:

- Ingredients: dates, almond butter, honey, chopped nuts
- Instructions: Fill dates with almond butter, honey, and chopped nuts.

Buffet:

Pasta Station:

- Ingredients: pasta, marinara sauce, roasted vegetables
- Instructions: Cook pasta according to package directions. Serve with marinara sauce and roasted vegetables.

Risotto Bar:

- Ingredients: Arborio rice, vegetable broth, sautéed onions and garlic

- Instructions: Cook Arborio rice with vegetable broth
and sautéed onions and garlic.

Stir-Fry Station:

- Ingredients: rice, mixed vegetables, stir-fry sauce
- Instructions: Cook rice and mixed vegetables
according to package directions. Serve with stir-fry
sauce.

Dessert Platters:

- Cookie Platter:

- Ingredients: vegan cookie dough
- Instructions: Preheat oven to 375°F (190°C). Scoop
vegan cookie dough onto a baking sheet and bake for
10-12 minutes.

- Fruit Platter:

- Ingredients: mixed fruit (e.g. grapes, berries, sliced
apples)
- Instructions: Arrange mixed fruit on the platter.

Champagne Toast:

- Ingredients: vegan champagne or sparkling cider

- Instructions: Pour vegan champagne or sparkling cider
into glasses and toast to the new year!

3. PLANT-BASED PARTY PLATTERS

1. CRUDITÉ PLATTER:

Arrange an assortment of fresh vegetables like carrots, celery, bell peppers, cucumbers, and cherry tomatoes on a platter, along with hummus, guacamole, or tahini dip for a colorful and healthy party snack.
A crudité platter is a great idea for a party snack! It's a light, refreshing, and healthy option that's perfect for a gathering. Here are some additional thoughts on how to make it even more appealing:

- Variety of vegetables: In addition to the ones you mentioned, consider adding other colorful vegetables like radishes, snap peas, and bell peppers.
- Dip options: Hummus, guacamole, and tahini are all great choices. You could also consider adding a tzatziki sauce or a spinach and artichoke dip for extra flavor.
- Garnishes: Add some fresh herbs like parsley, rosemary, or thyme to the platter for a pop of color and fragrance.

- Presentation: Arrange the vegetables in a visually appealing way, such as in a pattern or a rainbow-colored arrangement.
- Serving utensils: Provide small serving utensils like cocktail forks or toothpicks to make it easy for guests to grab a snack.

Here's a sample list of ingredients you could use for a crudité platter:

Vegetables:
- Carrots
- Celery
- Bell peppers
- Cucumbers
- Cherry tomatoes
- Radishes
- Snap peas

Dips:
- Hummus
- Guacamole
- Tahini
- Tzatziki sauce

- Spinach and artichoke dip

Garnishes:

- Fresh parsley

- Fresh rosemary

- Fresh thyme

Serving utensils:

- Cocktail forks

- Toothpicks

2. FRUIT PLATTER:

Create a beautiful display of sliced fruits such as strawberries, grapes, pineapple, melon, and kiwi on a platter, along with yogurt dip or chocolate sauce for dipping for a sweet and refreshing party treat.
A fruit platter is a great idea for a party treat! It's a light, refreshing, and healthy option that's perfect for a gathering. Here are some additional thoughts on how to make it even more appealing:

- Variety of fruits: In addition to the ones you mentioned, consider adding other colorful fruits like blueberries, raspberries, blackberries, and sliced peaches or nectarines.
- Yogurt dip: Offer a flavored yogurt dip like vanilla, strawberry, or mango to complement the fruits.
- Chocolate sauce: Provide a high-quality chocolate sauce for a sweet and indulgent treat.
- Garnishes: Add some fresh mint leaves or edible flowers like violas or pansies to the platter for a pop of color and fragrance.
- Presentation: Arrange the fruits in a visually appealing way, such as in a pattern or a rainbow-colored arrangement.

- Serving utensils: Provide small serving utensils like cocktail forks or skewers to make it easy for guests to grab a snack.

Here's a sample list of ingredients you could use for a fruit platter:

Fruits:

- Strawberries
- Grapes
- Pineapple
- Melon
- Kiwi
- Blueberries
- Raspberries
- Blackberries
- Sliced peaches or nectarines

Dips:

- Yogurt dip (vanilla, strawberry, or mango)
- Chocolate sauce

Garnishes:

- Fresh mint leaves

- Edible flowers (like violas or pansies)

Serving utensils:
- Cocktail forks
- Skewers

3. ANTIPASTO PLATTER:

Arrange a variety of marinated vegetables, olives, roasted nuts, and vegan cheeses on a platter, along with crusty bread or crackers for a delicious and elegant appetizer spread that's perfect for entertaining.

An antipasto platter is a great idea for entertaining! It offers a variety of flavors and textures that are easy to graze on. Here are some additional thoughts to make it even more appealing:

- Marinated vegetables: Consider using a mix of colorful vegetables like bell peppers, zucchini, cherry tomatoes, and eggplant, marinated in a herby Italian dressing.

- Olives: Add a selection of olives like Kalamata, green olives, and Castelvetrano for a salty, savory element.
- Roasted nuts: Roasted almonds, walnuts, or pistachios add a satisfying crunch.

- Vegan cheeses: Choose a variety of vegan cheeses like vegan mozzarella, vegan parmesan, and vegan gouda to provide a creamy element.

- Bread and crackers: Off crusty bread like baguette slices or crostini, and a variety of crackers like crostini or crudités.

- Garnishes: Add some fresh herbs like parsley, rosemary, or thyme to the platter for a pop of color and fragrance.

- Spreads: Consider adding some spreads like hummus, tapenade, or pesto to complement the antipasto selection.

Here's a sample list of ingredients you could use for an antipasto platter:

Marinated vegetables:
- Bell peppers
- Zucchini
- Cherry tomatoes
- Eggplant

Olives:
- Kalamata
- Green olives
- Castelvetrano

Roasted nuts:

- Almonds

- Walnuts

- Pistachios

Vegan cheeses:

- Vegan mozzarella

- Vegan parmesan

- Vegan gouda

Bread and crackers:

- Baguette slices

- Crostini

- Crackers

Garnishes:

- Fresh parsley

- Fresh rosemary

- Fresh thyme

Spreads:

- Hummus

- Tapenade

- Pesto

4. CHEESE BOARD:

Create a selection of vegan cheeses, crackers, fresh and dried fruits, nuts, and jams on a board for a sophisticated and indulgent party snack that will impress your guests. A cheese board is a great idea for a party snack! Vegan cheese options have come a long way in terms of taste and variety, and pairing them with complementary items like crackers, fruits, nuts, and jams creates a satisfying and elegant snack. Here are some suggestions to make your cheese board stand out:

Vegan cheeses:
   - Soft cheeses like vegan brie, feta, or goat cheese
   - Hard cheeses like vegan cheddar, parmesan, or gouda
   - Creamy cheeses like vegan mozzarella or burrata
- Crackers and bread:
   - Crostini or baguette slices
   - Crackers with seeds or nuts for added texture

Fresh fruits:
   - Grapes
   - Berries (strawberries, blueberries, raspberries)
   - Sliced apples or pears

Dried fruits:

- Cranberries

- Apricots

- Dates

Nuts:

- Almonds

- Walnuts

- Pistachios

Jams and spreads:

- Fruit jams (strawberry, blueberry, apricot)

- Nut butters (peanut butter, almond butter)

- Chocolate spreads (for a sweet and savory combination)

Remember to consider your guests' dietary restrictions and preferences when selecting items for your cheese board. You can also add garnishes like fresh herbs or edible flowers to make the board visually appealing.

5. DESSERT PLATTER:

Offer an assortment of bite-sized desserts like mini cupcakes, cookies, chocolate truffles, and fruit tarts on a platter for a sweet and irresistible ending to your party feast.

A dessert platter is a great way to end a party feast! Offering a variety of bite-sized desserts allows guests to sample a few different treats and satisfies their sweet tooth. Here are some suggestions to make your dessert platter shine:

Mini cupcakes:

- Vanilla, chocolate, or red velvet
- Decorated with colorful sprinkles or edible flowers
- Cookies:
- Chocolate chip, oatmeal raisin, or peanut butter
- Soft-baked or crispy, depending on your preference

Chocolate truffles:

- Made with dark, milk, or white chocolate
- Flavored with nuts, fruit, or spices for added depth
- Fruit tarts:
- Miniature pastry cups filled with fresh fruit curd

- Topped with a dollop of whipped cream or a sprinkle of powdered sugar

Consider adding a few extra touches to make your dessert platter special:

- Fresh fruit skewers or edible flowers for garnish
- Chocolate-dipped strawberries or bananas for a sweet and indulgent treat
- Macarons, mini eclairs, or other bite-sized pastries for added variety
- A small bowl of whipped cream or chocolate sauce for dipping

Remember to have fun and get creative with your dessert platter! It's a great way to showcase your culinary skills and leave a lasting impression on your guests.

CONCLUSION

As we reach the end of this culinary adventure, it's clear that embracing a plant-based lifestyle is so much more than just what's on our plates—it's a transformative journey that touches every aspect of our lives. From navigating social gatherings with confidence to championing sustainability and environmental stewardship, and from prioritizing our health and well-being to fostering a deeper sense of connection to the world around us, we've embarked on a path of growth, discovery, and positive change.

In the tapestry of life, each meal becomes a thread woven with intention and purpose—a delicious expression of our values, beliefs, and aspirations. With every bite of nourishing, plant-powered goodness, we're not just nourishing our bodies; we're nourishing our souls and contributing to a brighter, more compassionate world.

As we bid farewell to this cookbook, let's carry its lessons with us as we continue to savor the flavors of life, explore new culinary horizons, and cultivate a deeper sense of harmony with ourselves, each other, and the planet we call home. Here's to the journey ahead—a journey filled with abundance, vitality, and the boundless joy of living in alignment with our truest selves. Bon appétit, and may your plates be forever brimming with love, compassion, and the deliciousness of possibility.

TWO WEEKS MEAL PLANNING TABLE

WEEK ONE

Day	Mon	Tue	Wed	Thur	Fri	Sat	Sun
Bkft							
Lnch							
Dnr							
Snks							

WEEK TWO

Day	Mon	Tue	Wed	Thur	Fri	Sat	Sun
Bkft							
Lnch							
Dnr							
Snks